VIROLOGY RESEARCH PROGRESS

INFLUENZA AND RNA VIRUSES

EMERGENCE, CLASSIFICATION AND MANAGEMENT

VIROLOGY RESEARCH PROGRESS

Additional books in this series can be found on Nova's website under the Series tab.

Additional e-books in this series can be found on Nova's website under the e-book tab.

VIROLOGY RESEARCH PROGRESS

INFLUENZA AND RNA VIRUSES

EMERGENCE, CLASSIFICATION AND MANAGEMENT

ROXANNE H. BISHOP
EDITOR

NOVA BIOMEDICAL

New York

For permission to use material from this book please contact us:
Telephone 631-231-7269; Fax 631-231-8175
Web Site: http://www.novapublishers.com

LIBRARY OF CONGRESS CATALOGING-IN-PUBLICATION DATA

ISBN 978-1-63321-799-7
Library of Congress Control Number: 2014948046

Published by Nova Science Publishers, Inc. † New York

CONTENTS

PREFACE

In the spring of 2013, the influenza A (H7N9) virus shocked China, and caused 134 human infections with 45 deaths in its first influenza season. In the winter of 2013-2014, the virus struck China again and caused 273 cases with 108 deaths. This H7N9 outbreak has raised concern for another influenza pandemic. In this book, the epidemiology of the H7N9 outbreak, and the origin and diversity of the virus genome are discussed. This book examines the emergence and management of RNA viruses, like influenza, as well as the classifications of the viruses.

Although the majority of A(H1N1)pdm09 infections presents as a mild and self-limited disease, severe lung involvement has been responsible of high morbidity and mortality. Changes of binding affinity at the receptor binding site (RBS) play a critical role in viral tropism and virulence. Studies on viral correlates of disease severity identified that amino acid mutations in the haemagglutinin (HA) RBS are potentially responsible for outbreaks due to a switch in the receptor binding tropism leading to higher affinity for respiratory cells in the lower than in the upper respiratory tract and, therefore, a more aggressive disease. Specific HA mutations acquired during virus-host adaptation may enhance viral binding to α-2,3sialic acid receptors at the lower respiratory tract. HA-RBS sequence from codon 170 to 230 is essential for determining HA binding and is involved in antigen recognition. As described in Chapter 1, mutations at this point could alter antibody reactivity and viral tropism. Polymorphisms at the HA-RBS, such as G155E, S183P and D222G have been identified in animal models and confirmed in humans to increase viral affinity for the α-2,3 receptors and, thus, potentially associated with involvement of the lower respiratory tract.

During the 2009 A(H1N1)pdm09 outbreak, substitution of aspartic acid with glycine at position 222 (D222G) of HA1 subunit of A(H1N1)pdm09 has been associated with increased virulence, disease severity and fatal outcomes. To assess the contribution of HA-RBS variability in A(H1N1)pdm09 disease severity, a systematic review of Medline was performed for the presence of D222G and D222N polymorphisms in A(H1N1)pdm09 infection. Data on patient baseline characteristics, clinical and virological determinants were extracted and the association of D222G or D222N variants with severe disease was evaluated. Twenty-six published articles providing high quality data on both patients and virological determinants were retrieved, corresponding to 4,245 patients with A(H1N1)pdm09 infection in seasons 2009-2010 and 2010-2011.

Severe infection was reported for 1,335 patients (31%). D222G and D222N variants were described in 228 patients (5.4%) and A(H1N1)pdm09 HA substitutions D222G or N were harbored in a significantly higher proportion by patients with severe infection (15%) than by those with mild disease (0.9%, X^2 365.0, $p<0.0001$).

In conclusion, published data confirm the higher proportion of A(H1N1)pdm09 D222G and N variants in patients with severe disease. The study of A(H1N1)pdm09 correlates of disease severity, involving the detection of HA D222 variants at the receptor binding site, emphasizes the importance of a continuous monitoring of A(H1N1)pdm09 evolution for understanding virus-host interaction and adaptation.

To grasp the scientific information about cancer, its systematization is required. This systematization is conducted in the following succession, from general to particular: general theory of systems, theory of dissipative systems (synergetics), theory of life genesis based on hypercycles, and molecular biology.

In the context of such systematization, the process of cancerogenesis is scrutinized. Cancerogenesis is a process of continuous modification of gene expression in a cancerous cell due to epigenomic DNA methylation. The base of this process is one of the autocatalytic reactions as the simplest primary life form capable of replication, modification of species due to mutations, involving RNA reproduction of other cyclic reactions in the process, and competition with other replicative units. Such a reaction is referred to as hypercycle. On the one hand, this hypercycle ensures self-reproduction, on the other hand, epigenetic DNA reprogramming, which entails cancerous cell transformation. A hypercycle capable of such reprogramming is referred to as cancerogenic hypercycle.

A cancerogenic hypercycle is generated at the beginning as an autonomous process of RNA replication in the cell cytoplasm which has stopped the cooperation with DNA replication. Under the impact of diverse factors, it obtains the ability of concurring with the DNA replication, becomes the new organizer of order in the cell and, by and by, displaces and depresses the latter one (DNA replication). The condition for generation of a cancerogenic hypercycle is a hypercyclic link of two and more cyclic reactions based on common ferments and (or) on a RNA interference mechanism.

The generation of a cancerogenic hypercycle is also regarded as the generation of a new regressive dissipative system and the associated possibility of mathematical modelling and prognosticating of this process.

In Chapter 2, possible structures and forms of cancerogenic hypercycles are mentioned, the cancerous hyper-cycle based on interaction between RdRP and dsRNA resulting from this as a revision of the anti-tumour impact of the radiation and chemotherapy is scrutinized, as well as new possibilities of cancer diagnostic and treatment.

The difference concerning the approach to cancer treatment between the modern target therapy conception and the proposed conception is shown.

In the spring of 2013, the novel emerging influenza A (H7N9) virus has shocked China, and caused 134 human infections with 45 deaths in its first influenza season. In the winter of 2013-2014, the virus stroke China again and has caused 273 cases with 108 deaths (as of April 27th). The H7N9 outbreak has raised the concern of the next influenza pandemic. In Chapter 3, the authors briefly described the epidemiology of the H7N9 outbreak, and discussed the origin and diversity of the virus genome. Several models, including dynamic reassortments and genetic tuning models regarding the virus genesis, establishment and evolution were addressed. Moreover, the authors estimated and predicted the transmission routes of the H7N9 virus in China by means of big data. The co-circulation of H7N9 and varied subtypes of avian influenza viruses within poultry in China was described and discussed, as it is important for the establishment of the unpredictable HxNy influenza virus. Based on investigation of the molecular epidemiology of the H7N9 virus, the complete shutdown of the live poultry markets and firmly control of live poultry trade in China and Asian countries are called for to minimize avian influenza virus infections.

Currently global temperature change is a major aspect of climate changes so it is important to study how proteins of influenza A viruses adapt to temperature change because the understanding of this adaptation would help us to deal with influenza epidemics and pandemics. In order to get a whole picture on the adaptation in influenza A virus, the authors studied the adaptation of matrix protein 1 (M1) from influenza A virus to global temperature change. 2116 M1 proteins sampled from 1918 to October 2012 were converted by predictable portion and compared with the temperature changes (HadCRUT3v and CRUTEM4v data sets) in a 5° by 5° grid-box basis. Still, point-to-point comparisons were made from 1959 to 1998 in all and different species. In Chapter 4, the results showed that changes in temperatures and predictable portion of M1 proteins had similar trends during the period, highlighting impact of climate changes on influenza A viruses evolution.

Influenza A viruses, which are members of the orthomyxovirus family, cause epidemics and pandemics throughout the world. Recently, a novel swine-origin H1N1 influenza virus emerged, and human-to-human transmission of this virus led to the declaration of a pandemic by the World Health Organization (WHO) in 2009.

In addition, highly pathogenic H5N1 avian influenza viruses were detected in Hong Kong in 1997. Although the H5N1 viruses had not caused a pandemic until now, they could cause a pandemic at any time because mutations frequently occur in influenza viruses. Various approaches have been used to neutralize influenza viruses, such as anti-influenza virus drugs and vaccines.

Their main targets are hemagglutinin (HA) and neuraminidase (NA), two membrane proteins on the influenza virus that are major determinants of pathogenicity. It has been reported that HA and NA mutations occur frequently, which makes treating of influenza virus infections difficult. Although the authors can promptly analyze the DNA sequences of HA and NA genes derived from mutant viruses by using next-generation DNA sequencing technology, the DNA sequence does not provide functional information for the proteins encoded by the mutant DNAs. Such protein analyses are difficult because purification of the recombinant proteins includes burdensome steps. In Chapter 5, the authors introduce a new approach to solve this problem using a yeast cell surface engineering system. Using this system, it is possible to easily construct a comprehensive mutant protein library that is displayed on the yeast cell surface using the sequence of individual mutant DNAs, because the various inconvenient and troublesome steps of protein preparations can be avoided. In addition, it can be used to quickly evaluate whether the presently available drugs, such as oseltamivir and zanamivir, could be effective against the mutant proteins. HA- and NA-displaying yeasts can be targets for screening novel inhibitors in an available chemical library. In addition, the mutant proteins encoded by mutations that may occur in the future can be predictably prepared. The authors review the advantages of these approaches for influenza therapy.

Salivirus and klassevirus, possessing a positive-sense polyadenylated single-stranded RNA genome, are novel members of the family *Picornaviridae* and most closely related to Aichi virus of the genus *Kobuvirus*. Both salivirus and klassevirus were first described in 2009; salivirus was discovered in the feces of children with non-polio acute flaccid paralysis (AFP) in Nigeria (Stool Aichi-LIke virus), whereas klassevirus was found in the feces of children with gastroenteritis in the United States and Australia as well as in a sewage sample collected in Spain (Kobu-Like virus Associated with Stool and SEwage). Salivirus is genetically indistinguishable from klassevirus, and these viruses are currently classified into the novel genus, *Salivirus*. Salivirus/klassevirus has been identified in the feces of patients in Asian, European, and South American continents as well, suggesting its worldwide distribution. Recent studies also detected salivirus/klassevirus in wastewater, river water, and biosolids, in Asian, European, and American continents. As explained in Chapter 6, these recent findings have suggested that salivirus and klassevirus are emerging viral pathogens associated with gastroenteritis or non-polio AFP in infants and environmental transmission is likely. Further clinical and environmental studies are needed to better understand their prevalence, distribution, molecular epidemiology, and significance to public health.

In: Influenza and RNA Viruses
Editor: R. H. Bishop, pp. 1-23
ISBN: 978-1-63321-799-7

Chapter 1

UPDATE OF A(H1N1)PDM09 HAEMAGGLUTININ D222G AND D222N VARIANTS IN PATIENTS WITH SEVERE INFECTION

*Elisa Burdino, M.D.**, *Maria Grazia Milia, Tina Ruggiero and Valeria Ghisetti*
Laboratory of Microbiology and Virology,
Department of Infectious Diseases,
Amedeo di Savoia Hospital, Torino, Italy

Abstract

Although the majority of A(H1N1)pdm09 infections presents as a mild and self-limited disease, severe lung involvement has been responsible of high morbidity and mortality. Changes of binding affinity at the receptor binding site (RBS) play a critical role in viral tropism and virulence. Studies on viral correlates of disease severity identified that amino acid mutations in the haemagglutinin (HA) RBS are potentially responsible for outbreaks due to a switch in the receptor binding tropism leading to higher affinity for respiratory cells in the lower than in the upper respiratory tract and, therefore, a more aggressive disease. Specific HA mutations acquired during virus-host adaptation may enhance viral binding to α-2,3sialic acid receptors at the lower respiratory tract. HA-RBS sequence from

* E-mail address: elisa.burdino@libero.it; Tel. 00394393964; Fax. 00394393912 (Corresponding Author).

codon 170 to 230 is essential for determining HA binding and is involved in antigen recognition. Mutations at this point could alter antibody reactivity and viral tropism. Polymorphisms at the HA-RBS, such as G155E, S183P and D222G have been identified in animal models and confirmed in humans to increase viral affinity for the α-2,3 receptors and, thus, potentially associated with involvement of the lower respiratory tract.

During the 2009 A(H1N1)pdm09 outbreak, substitution of aspartic acid with glycine at position 222 (D222G) of HA1 subunit of A(H1N1)pdm09 has been associated with increased virulence, disease severity and fatal outcomes. To assess the contribution of HA-RBS variability in A(H1N1)pdm09 disease severity, a systematic review of Medline was performed for the presence of D222G and D222N polymorphisms in A(H1N1)pdm09 infection. Data on patient baseline characteristics, clinical and virological determinants were extracted and the association of D222G or D222N variants with severe disease was evaluated. Twenty-six published articles providing high quality data on both patients and virological determinants were retrieved, corresponding to 4,245 patients with A(H1N1)pdm09 infection in seasons 2009-2010 and 2010-2011.

Severe infection was reported for 1,335 patients (31%). D222G and D222N variants were described in 228 patients (5.4%) and A(H1N1)pdm09 HA substitutions D222G or N were harbored in a significantly higher proportion by patients with severe infection (15%) than by those with mild disease (0.9%, X^2 365.0, $p<0.0001$).

In conclusion, published data confirm the higher proportion of A(H1N1)pdm09 D222G and N variants in patients with severe disease. The study of A(H1N1)pdm09 correlates of disease severity, involving the detection of HA D222 variants at the receptor binding site, emphasizes the importance of a continuous monitoring of A(H1N1)pdm09 evolution for understanding virus-host interaction and adaptation.

1. Introduction

The most recent influenza pandemic, first recognized in Mexico in March 2009, has been caused by the novel 2009 influenza A H1N1 virus [A(H1N1) pdm09] containing a new combination of gene segments from swine and human viruses, as a result of multiple reassortment events over years that brought together in the same virus genomic segments from the classical swine H1N1 virus, the seasonal human H3N2, the North American avian and the Eurasian swine viruses [1].

Although the majority of A(H1N1)pdm09 infections presented as a mild and self-limited disease, severe pulmonary involvement requiring admission to Intensive Care Units (ICU) has been responsible of high morbidity and mortality. Apart from patients known to be at high risk for severe disease and complication (e.g., individuals with heart and renal conditions or asthma), A(H1N1)pdm09 gave rise to severe clinical condition in subjects without any underlying risk factor (e.g., pregnant women and young children) [1] with a final global toll of about 201,200 deaths due to severe respiratory disease [2]. For this reason, efforts to identify A(H1N1)pdm09 correlates of disease severity have been undertaken by the scientific community.

Changes of viral receptor binding affinity at the haemagglutinin (HA) receptor binding site (RBS) play a critical role in influenza virus tropism and virulence. Studies on viral correlates of disease severity identified that amino acid mutations in the HA receptor binding domain could be potentially responsible for influenza outbreaks due to a switch in the receptor binding tropism and a higher affinity for respiratory cells in the lower respiratory tract leading to a more aggressive disease [3].

The receptor binding site of HA is made of three structural elements: a 190-helix (residues 184–191), a 220-loop (residues 218–225), and a 130-loop (residues 131–135), while other highly conserved residues, (Tyr 91, Trp 150, His 180, and Tyr 192) form the inner pocket. Portions of RBS representing major antigenic sites include the conserved amino acid (aa) 192 and aa 184–191 in the 190-helix (Sb) and aa 222 in the 220-loop (Ca^{++}) (4). The receptor-binding specificity of avian and human influenza viruses is defined by amino acids exposed in the HA receptor-binding pocket. Human influenza viruses preferably attach to the sialic acid (SA) linked to a molecule of galactose by an α-2,6 linkage (SA α-2,6 Gal) that is only found on human epithelial cells located in the nasal mucosa, paranasal sinuses, pharynx, trachea and bronchi. On the contrary, avian viruses preferentially bind to SA α-2,3 Gal expressed on epithelial cells of the intestinal tract of waterfowl [5,6]. It is suggested that the A(H1N1) virus causing the Spanish Flu in 1918 could cross the species barrier between birds and humans thanks to HA mutations switching viral binding from avian to human cells [7]. Comparison of the avian HA consensus sequence with HA sequences from the 1918 virus demonstrates that they differed by only one or two of conserved residues (aa 187 and 222), depending on the viral isolate. In A(H1N1)pdm09 amino acids at HA positions 187 and 222 define the receptor binding specificity. HA-187D and HA-222D variants bind human-type receptors, whereas D187E and D222G variants shift the binding to avian-type receptors. In contrast to earlier assumptions, avian-type receptors are not restricted to birds, but they are also located on human epithelial cells lining the respiratory bronchiole and the alveolar walls. Their binding by viral variants whose tropism is switched, could, therefore, enable highly pathogenic influenza viruses to replicate in the lower respiratory tract [8].

In late November 2009, Norway researchers observed that the substitution of aspartic acid (D) with glycine (G) in A(H1N1)pdm09 HA glycoprotein subunit at position 222 (D222G), appeared with a significant frequency in severe and fatal human cases (5). Considering these and other observations, the World Health Organization (WHO) notified D222G substitution as a possible determinant of viral pathogenicity [9]. Moreover, D222G and other polymorphisms, such as G155E and S183P [4,10] have been identified in animal models, then confirmed in humans, to increase viral affinity for the α-2,3 receptors and thus, potentially associated with involvement and infection of the lower respiratory tract. Findings of a novel A(H1N1)pdm09 subclade in America suggested that also the D222N variant was correlated with severe clinical manifestation [11].

Investigations on D222G and D222N mutations resulted in an increasing number of reports [12], the majority of them agreeing that D222G variants were mainly found in severe disease: 8.7% in Finland [13], 6.2% in Scotland [14], 5% and 37.5% in Spain [15,16], 8.3% in France [17], 43.5%, 5.8%, 4.3%, 11.1% 29% and 37.5% in Italy [6,18–22], 41% in Germany [8], 16% in Greece [23], 4.8% in Tunisia [24], 14.3% in China [25], 11.6% in USA [26], 24% in Mexico [27], 4.1%, 21% and 17.4% in Hong Kong [28–30], 15.4% in India [31], 20% in Australia [32] and 10% in Japan [33]. Understanding the association of D222G and D222N variants with a more virulent and pathogenic A(H1N1)pdm09 phenotype is critical to improve the understanding of virus-host interaction and the management of A(H1N1)pdm09 infection [5,14,30].

2. Search Strategy: Study Evaluation and Data Extraction

To assess the contribution of HA-RBS variability in A(H1N1)pdm09 disease severity, a systematic review of Medline from January 2009 to November 2013 for A(H1N1)pdm09 D222G variants was performed.

Epidemiological studies (clinical reports, case-control and cohort studies) including genetic study of A(H1N1)pdm09 pandemic from March 2009 (corresponding to the first pandemic wave in Mexico) to April 2011 [A(H1N1)pdm09 pandemic and post-pandemic period] were included. The association between disease severity and HA mutations at 222 codon, in particular D222G or D222N variants, was investigated. Only articles reporting results on both the presence of HA-222 mutations in viral strains and patient clinical outcomes were included. Selected studies included subjects of all ages and sex, with or without risk factor for A(H1N1)pdm09 disease severity, inpatients, outpatients and subjects from the surveillance influenza networks, for whom a clinical and laboratory diagnosis of A(H1N1)pdm09 was performed. Outcome measures were severe conditions related to infection by strains of A(H1N1)pdm09 characterized by presence of HA mutation at codon D222.

Medline, PubMed central, WHO regional, national and international indexes were searched. Keywords including *H1N1 pandemic influenza* OR *influenza A(H1N1)* AND D222G/N mutation at the HA gene [including "*HA mutation in pandemic influenza A(H1N1) virus* OR *D222G/N mutation*"] were used. Title, abstract and full text were screened according to "*disease severity* OR *critical care/intensive care* OR *severe/fatal cases*" following WHO and Zarychansky criteria [34,35] and the recommendations for Preferred Reporting Items for Systematic Reviews and Meta-Analyses (PRISMA) [36].

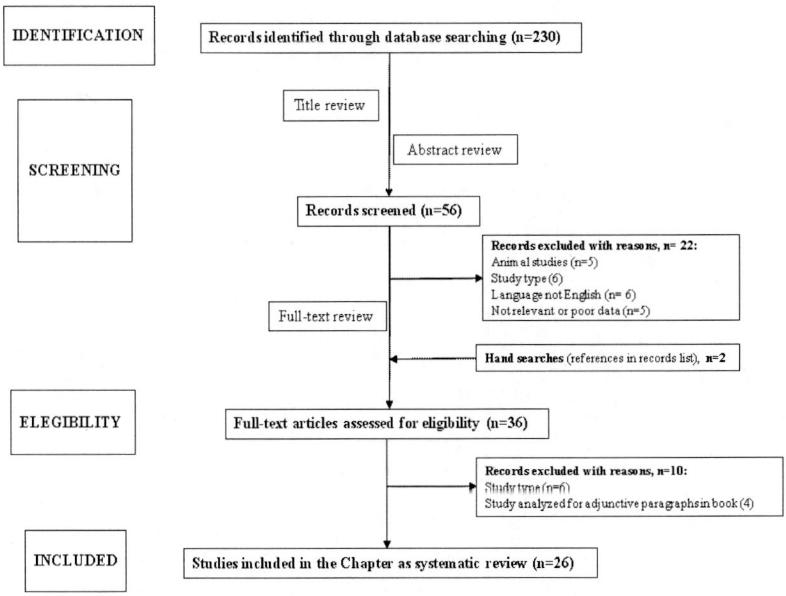

Figure 1. Flowchart for Chapter selection process.

Two hundred and thirty records were retrieved, but only 56 full-text articles were relevant to the aim; 26 articles providing high quality data on both patients and virologic determinants (Figure 1) [5,6,8,12–17,19–33,37,38] were considered eligible, corresponding to 13,112 patients with A(H1N1)pdm09 influenza in the two seasons 2009-2010 and 2010-2011. Genetic determinants of A(H1N1)pdm09 were available for 4,245 viral strains, (4,245 patients), 1,335 with severe

Table 1. Summary of the characteristics of the studies considered for inclusion

References	Patient (pt) study group	N. of viral strains genotyped on HA-RBS			Identified HA-222 variants (*N. of viral strains*, %)			
					Mild disease		Severe disease	
		Total	Mild disease	Severe disease	D222G*	D222N	D222G*	D222N
Melidou et al. [23]	Hospitalized pts	44	13	31	2 (15.4%)	0	5 (16%)	0
Ikonen et al. [13]	Hospitalized and ICU pts	134	111	23	0	0	2 (8.7%)	0
Rykkvin et al. [12]	Outpatients and hospitalized pts	459**	381	78	0	1(0.3%)	13 (16.7%)	3 (3.8%)
Kilander et al. (5)	Hospitalized pts	266	205	61	0	1 (0.5%)	11 (18%)	3 (4.9%)
Alonso et al. [37]	Hospitalized pts	29	13	16	0	0	0	0
Ledesma et al. [15]	Outpatients and hospitalized pts	806	533	273	0	0	14 (5%)	2 (0.7%)
Anton et al. [16]	Outpatients and hospitalized pts	189	181	8	0	0	3 (37.5 %)	0
Malato et al. [17]	Hospitalized and ICU pts	24	0	24	0	0	2(8.3%)	0
Miller et al. [14]	Outpatients and hospitalized pts	58	26	32	0	0	2 (6.2%)	2 (6.2%)
Wedde et al. [8]	Outpatients and hospitalized pts	357	258	99	0	2 (0.8%)	41 (41%)	0
Baldanti et al. [18]	Outpatients, hospitalized and ICU pts	131	108	23	2 (1.8%)	0	10 (43.5%)	0
Puzzelli et al. [20]	Outpatients and hospitalized pts	169	117	52	1 (0.9%)	0	3 (5.8%)	0
Puzzelli et al. [19]	Outpatients and hospitalized pts	130	107	23	0	0	1 (4.3 %)	0
Ruggiero et al. [21]	Outpatients, hospitalized and ICU pts	102	78	24	1 (1.3%)	1 (1.3)	7 (29%)	1 (4.2%)
Piralla et al. [6]	Outpatients, hospitalized and ICU pts	139	94	45	0	0	5 (11.1%)	3 (6.7%)
Vazquez-Perez et al. [27]	Outpatients, hospitalized and ICU pts	77	27	50	0	0	12 (24%)	1 (2%)

References	Patient (pt) study group	N. of viral strains genotyped on HA-RBS			Identified HA-222 variants (*N. of viral strains*, %)			
					Mild disease		Severe disease	
		Total	Mild disease	Severe disease	D222G*	D222N	D222G*	D222N
Potdar et al. [31]	Hospitalized pts	13	0	13	0	0	2 (15.4%)	0
Wang et al. [32]	Outpatients, hospitalized and ICU pts	127	97	30	11 (11.3%)	0	6 (20%)	1 (3.3%)
Nakajima et al. [33]	Fatal pts	10	0	10	0	0	1 (10%)	0
Mak et al. [30]	Outpatients and hospitalized pts	458	239	219	0	1 (0.4%)	9 (4.1%)	3 (1.4%)
Chan et al. [28]	Hospitalized pts	63	40	23	0	0	4 (17.4%)	1 (4.3%)
Wu et al. [25]	Outpatients and hospitalized pts	223	195	28	1 (0.5%)	0	4 (14.3%)	2 (7.1%)
Chen et al. [29]	Hospitalized pts	117	60	57	0	1 (1.7%)	12 (21%)	1 (1.7%)
Selleri et al. [22]	Hospitalized pts	27	19	8	0	0	3 (37.5%)	0
DeVries et al. [26]	Fatal pts	43	0	43	0	0	5 (11.6%)	0
Moussi et al. [24]	Outpatients and hospitalized pts	50	8	42	1 (12.5%)	0	2 (4.8%)	0

* Included "mixed quasispecies", for details see Table 2 and Table 2a.

** Total number: 462, but 3 patients with clinical outcome unknown were excluded from total.

A(H1N1)pdm09 infection and 2,910 with mild disease. Table 1 shows characteristics of selected studies. All studies were retrospectively focused on the association of genetic A(H1N1)pdm09 determinant and severe disease compared to mild one. For the definition of the influenza severe disease, above mentioned criteria [34,35] were followed by all Authors, while in the definition of "mild" disease, patients with "*non severe*" or "*uncomplicated*" influenza and individuals from national and local surveillance systems were included.

Statistical analysis was performed using PASW Statistics 18.0.2 (SPSS Inc, Chicago, IL, USA). Analysis of mutation frequencies within different groups of patients was performed using the chi square test and considered to be significant at a level of 0.05.

3. Frequency of D222G and D222N Variants in Severe and Mild A(H1N1)pdm09 Disease

Twenty-six studies combining epidemiological and virological data from worldwide patients with A(H1N1)pdm09 infection were analyzed to determine the worldwide frequency of D222G and D222N mutants in severe infection in comparison with mild disease. Table 1 shows main characteristics of the selected studies, summing up to 4,245 patients for whom D222 wild-type or variants were available. Severe infection was reported for 1,335 patients (31%). D222G and D222N variants were described in 228 patients (5.4%) and were harbored in a significantly higher proportion by viral strains infecting patients with severe disease (15%, 202 patients) while they were only sporadically found in patients with mild conditions (0.9%, corresponding to 26 patients, X^2 365.0, $p<0.0001$). As a consequence, D222 wild-type or D222E variant, which are known for not being associated with severe disease [22], were present in a significantly higher proportion in patients with mild A(H1N1)pdm09 disease (n=2,884) compared with those affected by severe condition (n=1,133). Table 2 and 2a show the prevalence of D222G and D222N variants and HA-222 quasispecies. D222G variants were reported in 6.4% (n=86) and 0.24% (n=7) of patients with severe and mild condition, respectively. D222N mutants were less represented than D222G accounting for only 1.7% of strains in severe disease (0.24% in mild infection), while HA-222 quasispecies were mostly reported in severe disease (7% vs. 0.4% in mild condition) (Table 2a). Therefore, harboring D222G or D222N variants were associated with a significant high risk of severe infection (odds ratio 19.79, 95% CI 13.07-29.93). This data are in agreement with those from the European Centre for Disease Prevention and Control (ECDC) [1] and WHO that reported in the year 2010, the presence of D222G mutation in at least 20 countries, affecting from 1.8% of patients with mild disease to 7.1% of patients with severe condition [9].

Table 2. Frequency of HA-222 variants in mild and severe disease

HA-222 variants	Mild disease *N. of strains* (Total n. 2,910)	Severe disease *N. of strains* (Total n. 1,335)	Total *N. of strains* (n. 4,245)
D222D (wild-type)	2,610 (89.7%)	1,025 (76.8%)	3,635 (85.6%)
D222E	274 (9.4%)	108 (8.1%)	382 (9%)
Total	**2,884 (99.1%)**	**1,133 (85%)**	**4,017 (94.6%)**
HA-222 variants known to be associated with severe disease			
D222G	7 (0.24%)	86 (6.4%)	93 (2.2%)
HA-222 quasispecies *	12 (0.4%)	93 (7%)	105 (2.5%)
D222N	7 (0.24%)	23 (1.7%)	30 (0.7%)
Total	**26 (0.9%)****	**202 (15%)****	**228 (5.4%)**

* Including D222D/G, D222G/E, D222G/A, D222D/G/N, D222G/N and D222D/G/N/E/A/S/V/Y (see details in Tab 2a).

** X^2 365.0, p<0.0001.

Table 2a. HA-222 quasispecies in mild and severe disease

HA-222 quasispecies	Mild disease *N. of strains (%)*	Severe disease *N. of strains (%)*	Total *N. of strains (%)*
D222D/G	1(8.3%)	59 (63.4%)	60 (57%)
D222G/E	1 (8.3%)	3 (3.2%)	4 (3.8%)
D222G/A D222D/G/N	0 1/12 (8.3%)	1 (1.1%) 11 (11.8%)	1 (1%) 12 (11.4%)
D222G/N	0	2 (2.2%)	2 (2%)
D222D/G/N/E/A/S/V/Y	9/12 (75%)	17 (18.3%)	26 (24.8)
Total	**12 (11.4%)**	**93 (88.6%)**	**105**

4. Molecular Methods for the Detection of A(H1N1)pdm09 D222G and D222N Variants

To determine the genetic variability at nucleotide positions 715–716 of HA open reading frame coding for amino acid 222, two different strategies of nucleic acid sequencing were use in the selected articles: the classical Sanger direct nucleic acid sequencing and, more recently, "next generation sequencing" (NGS) methods.

In studies published between the year 2012 and 2013, NGS technologies allowed the identification of HA-222 variability at the level of quasispecies due to their significantly higher sensitivity than the Sanger method. In fact, the conventional Sanger technique used by the majority of studies may lead to a general underestimation of D222 variants and the reason is that standard population-based DNA sequencing does not allow to appreciate the composition of viral population at a quasispecies level, that is minor variants can be detected only if they represent a proportion higher than 15-20% of the whole population. A recent work [8] outlined a much higher detection rate of variants at position 222 with ultra-deep pyrosequencing (UDPS) that found G and N variants in >40% of patients compared to <19% with standard population-based DNA sequencing. Other studies [12,38] have demonstrated that with UDPS or clonal analysis it is possible to find these variants not only in samples from the lower respiratory tract, but also in samples from the upper respiratory one and that the proportion of upper respiratory samples carrying D222 variants increases to levels similar to those of the lower tract. Therefore, discrepancy in findings from different studies must take into account the different sensitivity of methods applied for viral detection and typing [12,22].

Other critical aspect is that when A(H1N1)pdm09 sequences are obtained from viral strains after cell-culturing rather than directly from clinical specimens, genetic changes may have been selected during the growth in cell culture systems. Therefore, WHO recommendations [9] for A(H1N1)pdm09 specimens testing state that the direct evaluation of clinical specimens is much more reliable for molecular analysis, including nucleic acid sequencing at HA position 222, than viral typing from cell culture. Other WHO recommendations are: (i) to obtain multiple, serial respiratory specimens in the early stage of illness and prior to the administration of antiviral therapy, and (ii) that paired clinical specimens from both the upper and lower respiratory tract should be obtained whenever possible, especially for critically ill patients.

The evaluation of the presence of multiple viral variants within the same patient but from different body compartments showed that polymorphisms are not limited to position 222, but may involve other HA segments, supporting the hypothesis of intra-host viral evolution and adaptation. The presence of multiple D222 variants in the same patient has been found in fifteen studies [8,12–15,17,22,23,26–29,32,33,38], some of them also reporting other poorly known D222 variants such as D222Y and D222A [13,15].

Implications of these findings are of great interest from both a pathogenic and epidemiological standpoint, as they suggest that the emergence and predominance of more aggressive variants may be the result of a single-patient-dependent phenomenon. Rykkvin et al. [12] and Wedde et al. [8] underlined that D222 variants could be detected as double peaks by the conventional Sanger method and that D222D/G quasispecies was more frequent in fatal (73%) and hospitalized (59%) patients than in community ones (33%). In Selleri et al. [22], variants carrying D222G or D222N were detected as minority components of the viral quasispecies with an amplicon-based UDPS approach. With this technique, D222E variants appeared to be the most frequent one in both severe and moderate–mild patients, confirming the lack of association between D222E and disease severity, that was on the contrary, previously reported [5]. HA-222 quasispecies were also identified by Wang et al. [32] who reported mixture of D/N/G/S in patients with both severe and mild infection by direct sequencing and clonal analysis.

5. Detection of A(H1N1)pdm09 D222G and D222N Variants in Upper and Lower Respiratory Tract

Substitutions at position D222, located in the HA-RBS cavity at the Ca^{++} antigenic site, can change RBS properties from acid and polar to neutral and non-polar, altering viral tropism. A(H1N1)pdm09 HA D222G mutation has been identified as a potential virulence marker because it is responsible of the above mentioned changes including a receptor switch allowing for viral invasion of the lower respiratory system. To understand the role of D222G and HA-222 quasispecies in worsening clinical condition of A(H1N1)pdm09 infection it is important to understand the presence of these variants in different compartments of the upper and lower respiratory tract.

Limitation for the comprehension of D222 variants prevalence and their role in lower respiratory tract infection is that in the majority of published studies, samples from the lower respiratory tract were available only in a minority of them (bronchoalveolar lavage were obtained in only 10.8% of patients) as well as that matched upper and lower respiratory samples could not be tested in most of the

Table 3. Molecular Methods for the detection of HA-222 variants

References	Methods	HA-222 variants (N. of viral strain identified)	Detection of HA-222 quasispecies (yes/no)
Melidou et al. [23]	Direct sequencing	D222G (n=4), D222D/G (n=3)	yes
Ikonen et al. [13]	Direct sequencing	D222D/G (n=2), D222D/Y (n=1)	yes
Rykkvin et al. [12]	Direct sequencing + Pyrosequencing	D222G (n=2), D222D/G (n=7), D222G/E (n=2), D222G/N (n=1), D222D/G/N (n=1), D222N (n=4)	yes
Kilander et al. [5]	Direct sequencing	D222G (n=11), D222N (n=4)	no
Alonso et al. [37]	Direct sequencing	D222G (n=0)	no
Ledesma et al. [15]	Direct sequencing	D222G (n=11), D222D/G (n=2), D222G/A (n=1), D222N (n=2)	yes
Anton et al. [16]	Direct sequencing	D222G (n=3)	no
Malato et al. 17]	Direct sequencing	D222G (n=1), D222E/G (n=1)	yes
Miller et al. [14]	Direct sequencing	D222G (n=1), D222D/G (n=1), D222N (n=2)	yes
Wedde et al. [8]	Direct sequencing + Pyrosequencing	D222G (n=4), D222D/G (n=30), D222D/G/N/V/Y (n=5), D222D/G/N (n=2), D222N (n=2)	yes
Baldanti et al. [18]	Direct sequencing	D222G (n=6), D222D/G (n=3), D222E/G (n=1), D222D/G/N (n=2)	yes
Puzzelli et al. [20]	Direct sequencing	D222G (n=4)	no
Puzzelli et al. [19]	Direct sequencing	D222G (n=1)	no

References	Methods	HA-222 variants (N. of viral strain identified)	Detection of HA-222 quasispecies (yes/no)
Ruggiero et al. [21]	Direct sequencing	D222G (n=8), D222N (n=2)	no
Piralla et al. [6]	Direct sequencing	D222G (n=5), D222N (n=3)	no
Vazquez-Perez et al. [27]	Direct sequencing + Illumina	D222G (n=3), D222D/G (n=5), D222D/G//N/E (n=4), D222N (n=1)	yes
Potdar et al. [31]	Direct sequencing	D222G (n=2)	no
Wang et al. [32]	Direct sequencing + Clonal analysis	D222D/G (n=1), D222D/G/N/S (n=16), D222 N (n=1)	yes
Nakajima et al. [33]	Direct sequencing + Clonal analysis	D222G/N (n=1)	yes
Mak et al. [30]	Direct sequencing	D222G (n=9), D222N (n=4)	no
Chan et al. [28]	Direct sequencing	D222G (n=2), D222D/G (n=1), D222D/G/N (n=1), D222N (n=1)	yes
Wu et al. [25]	Direct sequencing	D222G (n=5), D222N (n=2)	no
Chen et al. [29]	Direct sequencing + Clonal analysis	D222G (n=7), D222D/G (n=4), D222D/G/N (n=1), D222N (n=2)	yes
Selleri et al. [22]	Direct sequencing + UDPS-454	D222D/G (n=1), D222D/G//N (n=1), D222D/G//N/E/A (n=1)	yes
DeVries et al. [26]	Direct sequencing + Pyrosequencing	D222G (n=1), D222D/G/N (n=4)	yes
Moussi et al. [24]	Direct sequencing	D222G (n=3)	no

studies. Only in ten articles, the prevalence of HA D222 variants could be evaluated in matched lower and upper airway specimens from the same patients (Table 4), corresponding to 56 patients for whom matched samples were available [5,6,12,19,21,28,29,32,33,38]. In these studies, D222G variants were detected in samples from both the upper and the lower respiratory tract, with a slightly higher prevalence in those from the lower respiratory airways. Interestingly, HA substitution D222N was present only in specimens from the lower respiratory tract, being much less frequent than D222G. Wild-type D222 or D222E (D and E have the same polarity) predominated in specimens from the upper respiratory tract (68%) and significantly diminished in those from the lower one. The proportion of D222G and HA-222 quasispecies was generally higher in the lower than in the upper airway (55% vs. 32%) suggesting that D222G may be present in both upper and lower respiratory airways, even if they preferentially segregate in the lower respiratory tract, where increased virus replication and higher virus load have also been shown [38].

The viral wild-type population interacts more efficiently with α-2,6 receptors, whereas D222G and D222N variants are characterized by expanded tropisms, binding α-2,3 receptors, highly represented in the lower respiratory tract. Consequently, mutated viruses can induce infection at that level, increasing the clinical severity of influenza infection. The predominance of D222G strains in the lower respiratory tract strengthens the hypothesis of their fitness in this biological environment. The frequent detection of mixtures of viral variants at this level supports the hypothesis of an intra-host evolution of D222G and D222N variants in individual patients, as opposed to their spreading within the population. In other words, the emergence of quasispecies variability at residue 222 might be a dynamic event during the course of the infection, rather than representing the stable detection of a completely changed D222G residue. This is also supported by the longer illness duration of severe and fatal cases, due to the time lapse required by the selection of genetic variants that best fit into the lower respiratory tract environment. A low capability of mutated variants to inter-human spread might also account for the reduced circulation of D222G and D222N variants and the mild clinical impact of the A(H1N1)pdm09 pandemic [8]. Taken together, these data confirm that viruses with a D222G or D222N substitutions exhibit an altered tropism that accompanies viral progression into the lower airways.

Table 4. HA-222 variants in matched upper and lower respiratory specimens

References		Detection of HA-222 variants *(N. of strains)*							
		From Upper Respiratory Specimens				From Lower Respiratory Specimens			
		D222D (WT) and D222E	**D222G**	**D222 N**	**HA-222 quasispecies**	**D222D (WT) and D222E**	**D222G**	**D222N**	**HA-222 quasispecies**
Baldanti et al.[18] Chen et al. [29] Wang et al. [32] Kilander et al. [5] Puzzelli et al. [19] Chan et al. [28] Nakajima et al.[33] Rykkvin et al.[12] Ruggiero et al. [21] Piralla et al. [6]	**2009-2010-2011**	D222D (n=34) D222E (n=5)	D222G (n=10)	ND*	D222D/N (n=1) D222E/D (n=1) D222D/G/N/S (n=2) D222D/G (n=1) D222G/N (n=1) D222D/G (n=2)	D222D (n=23) D222E (n=3)	D222G (n=14)	D222N (n=3)	D222D/G/N (n=2) D222E/D (n=1) D222D/G (n=6) D222G/N (n=2) D222D/G/N/S (n=2) D222E/G (n=1)
	Total *N.*	n=39 (68%)	n=10 (18%)		n=8 (14%)	n=26 (45%)	n=14 (25%)	n=3 (5%)	n=14 (25%)
			32%				55%		

* ND: not detected.

6. Viral Evolution of A(H1N1)pdm09 D222G and D222N Variants

Influenza A(H1N1)pdm09 has emerged following a recent reassortment between swine strains and jump into the human population has been tentatively dated at the beginning of the year 2009. Since the early times, the history the new virus lead us to appreciate its differentiation in clades [39].

Valli et al. [39] demonstrated that A(H1N1)pdm09 shifted from an initial mixed clade pattern to the predominance of one clade (clade 7) during the course of the pandemic. Clade 7 originated in late March 2009 and appeared in New York a few weeks after clades 1 and 2 were isolated in Mexico and California, but all viral clades were reported to co-circulate in all continents [39]. In most European countries, different clades were co-circulating in the first pandemic months, when the great majority of the infections were imported by travelers (mostly from North and South America) who had become infected abroad. A second, more intense wave occurred during the period October-November 2009. Unlike the first epidemic, the second peak was characterized by clade 7 (circulating at low intensity during the whole summer) rapid spread in children and young adults due to the opening of schools, kindergartens and other communities after the summer holiday. While in the Southern hemisphere (Oceania and South America) clade 7 was already predominant by the end of April 2009, reflecting perhaps the spread of the epidemic in the Southern part of the globe during winter season, in Singapore, China and Scandinavian countries the shift occurred later, between June and July. The hypothesis that clade 7 is characterized by a selective advantage, in terms of transmission over other clades is intriguing, but has yet to be demonstrated.

Important observations can be inferred by molecular and phylogenetic analysis of A(H1N1)pdm09 strains. Table 5 shows the comparison of total or partial HA sequences from A(H1N1)pdm09 isolated with the A/California/07/2009 (H1N1) strain as reference. The majority of authors [5,6,13,20,21,23,25,31,39–43] agreed that D222G and D222N sporadically appeared in phylogenetically distant viruses, with very limited cluster transmission [42]. In fact, D222G spread into very few clusters as reported by Piralla et al. [6], Wu et al. [25] and Ruggiero et al. [21]. In agreement with the rare circulation of these mutants during periods of high spread of influenza, phylogenetic analysis by Ruggiero et al. [21] identified only two small clusters of D222G viruses, one due to the nosocomial spread of a D222G variant and both including ICU admitted patients requiring advanced respiratory support. Therefore, the high frequency of

D222G strains in critically ill patients could be explained by the selection of these mutants in the context of disease severity at the individual level instead of viral spreading.

Among other HA-RBS substitutions associated with severe disease, the most significantly reported was the mutation S183P, shared by all 1918 H1N1 viruses. Ruggiero et al. [21] identified S183P in 2011 circulating strains from 10 inpatients, two of them dying of A(H1N1)pdm09 complications. S183P was associated with D222G in 2 patients with severe disease and absent or alone in those with mild disease. Analysis of European A(H1N1)pdm09 strains identified only another virus carrying the double mutations S183P and D222G from a patient who died in the year 2010 in England. Therefore, it is possible that the rare combination of the double mutant S183P and D222G characterizes a more virulent strain.

Table 5. Studies including molecular methods for D222G phylogenesis and cluster analysis

References	N. of strains studied	D222G cluster detection Yes/No	Other HA polymorphisms associated with severe disease
Melidou et al. [23]	44	Yes (1 cluster)	Q293H
Ikonen et al. [13]	141	No	None
Rykkvin et al. [12]	462	No	None
Falcone et al. [40]	NA*	No	None
Puzzelli et al. [19]	130	Yes (1 cluster)	G155E
Valli et al. [39]	42	No	None
Valli et al. [41]	2492	Yes (2 cluster)	None
Ruggiero et al. [21]	2704	Yes (2 cluster)	S183P
Piralla et al. [6]	163	No	R205K, I216V, V249L
Zehender et al. [42]	5844	No	None
Potdar et al. [31]	698	No	None
Wu et al. [25]	223	No	None
El Moussi et al. [43]	NA*	No	None

* NA: not available.

Melidou et al. [23] reported that in severe A(H1N1)pdm09 infections in Greece, viral strains clustered in the same clade, sharing the mutation Q293H. The association of Q293H with increased disease severity was also confirmed by a report from Brazil [3]. Piralla et al. [6] observed the simultaneous circulation of four A(H1N1)pdm09 clusters in an highly populated area including approximately one sixth of the total Italian population. Among these clusters, one was characterized by mutations R205K, I216V and V249L and about 70% of patients infected with this variant developed complications and severe infection.

7. Conclusion

Worldwide surveillance studies on pandemic influenza have reported that A(H1N1)pdm09 infection is associated with a higher risk of severe disease, hospitalization and ICU admission than seasonal influenza. The natural tendency of influenza viruses to acquire point mutations at different genomic positions is very well known and changes at the receptor binding site can alter antigenic properties and viral pathogenicity. Data selected from published studies referring to A(H1N1)pdm09 worldwide surveillance (from May 2009 to April 2011) and reporting viral genetic determinants in association with severe disease, identified mutations and substitutions at position 222 (either as G or N) in a significantly higher proportion of patients with severe disease (15%) than in patients with mild infection (0.9%). The increased virulence of D222G and D222N strains is postulated due to enhanced binding affinity for the α-2,3 sialic acid receptor present at higher density on cell surface in the lower respiratory tract rather than the α-2,6 sialic acid receptor located on upper respiratory cells, supporting the hypothesis that viruses with dual receptor binding specificity can replicate at high level in lung tissue producing a more aggressive disease. In agreement with the rare circulation of these mutants during periods of high spread of influenza virus circulation, clusters of virus harboring these variants very rarely occurred. The high frequency of D222G and D222N variants in critically ill patients could be explained by the selection of these mutants in the context of disease severity at the individual level instead of viral spreading.

Important limitations for a full comprehension of the prevalence of D222 mutants and their role in A(H1N1)pdm09 lower respiratory disease, are that lower respiratory samples were available only in a minority of studies as well as that matched upper and lower respiratory samples could not be analysed in order to understand the distribution of D222 variants. Therefore, the presence of D222G and D222N variants can certainly be underestimated, even if there are evidences of these variants in the upper respiratory tract [8,22]. Underestimation may also be due to the sensitivity of the technique applied for viral genotyping, that is, in the majority of the studies, conventional Sanger DNA sequencing that does not allow appreciating the composition of viral population at a quasispecies level. In fact, a much higher detection rate of D222 variants has been found by NGS techniques that are much more sensitive than conventional DNA sequencing ones [22]. Nevertheless, all the studies showed a general agreement that D222G and D222N variants could be mostly detected in patients with severe A(H1N1)pdm09 disease.

Finally, infections with mixed HA-222 viral populations as frequently reported by the application of ultrasensitive techniques may play a critical role in disease severity. It is important to emphasize that a poor clinical prognosis is strongly associated with the presence of a quasispecies mixtures at this residue.

In conclusion, the study of A(H1N1)pdm09 viral correlates of disease severity, involving the detection of HA variants at the receptor binding site, underlines the importance of a continuous monitoring of A(H1N1)pdm09 genetic evolution and that D222G and D222N variants have certainly a major role in in disease severity. These data strongly support the epidemiologic surveillance of strain circulation for understanding virus-host interaction, adaptation and viral correlates of disease severity.

References

[1] Simonsen, L; Spreeuwenberg, P; Lustig, R; Taylor, RJ; Fleming, DM; Kroneman, M; et al. Global mortality estimates for the 2009 Influenza Pandemic from the GLaMOR project: a modeling study. *PLoS Med.*, 2013, 10, e1001558.

[2] Dawood, FS; Iuliano, AD; Reed, C; Meltzer, MI; Shay, DK; Cheng, P-Y; et al. Estimated global mortality associated with the first 12 months of 2009 pandemic influenza A H1N1 virus circulation: a modelling study. *Lancet Infect Dis.*, 2012, 12, 687–95.

[3] Glinsky, G V. Genomic analysis of pandemic (H1N1) 2009 reveals association of increasing disease severity with emergence of novel hemagglutinin mutations. *Cell cycle.*, 2010, 9, 958–70.

[4] Nunthaboot, N; Rungrotmongkol, T; Malaisree, M; Kaiyawet, N; Decha, P; Sompornpisut, P; et al. Evolution of human receptor binding affinity of H1N1 hemagglutinins from 1918 to 2009 pandemic influenza A virus. *J Chem Inf Model.*, 2010, 23, 50, 1410–7.

[5] Kilander, A; Rykkvin, R; Dudman, SG; Hungnes, O. Observed association between the HA1 mutation D222G in the 2009 pandemic influenza A(H1N1) virus and severe clinical outcome, Norway 2009-2010. *Eurosurveill.*, 2010, 4, 15, 1–3.

[6] Piralla, A; Pariani, E; Rovida, F; Campanini, G; Muzzi, A; Emmi, V; et al. Segregation of virulent influenza A(H1N1) variants in the lower respiratory

tract of critically ill patients during the 2010-2011 seasonal epidemic. *PLoS One.*, 2011, 6, e28332.

[7] Ellis, J; Galiano, M; Pebody, R; Lackenby, A; Thompson, C; Bermingham, A; et al. Virological analysis of fatal influenza cases in the United Kingdom during the early wave of influenza in winter 2010/11. *Eurosurveill.*, 2011, 16, 1–6.

[8] Wedde, M; Wählisch, S; Wolff, T; Schweiger, B. Predominance of HA-222D/G Polymorphism in Influenza A(H1N1)pdm09 Viruses Associated with Fatal and Severe Outcomes Recently Circulating in Germany. *PLoS One.*, 2013, 8: e57059.

[9] World Health Organization. Preliminary review of D222G amino acid substitution in the haemagglutinin of pandemic influenza A (H1N1) 2009 viruses. *Wkly Epidemiol Rec.*, 2010, 85, 21–8.

[10] Ilyushina, N; Khalenkov, AM; Seiler, JP; Forrest, HL; Bovin, NV; Marjuki, H; et al. Adaptation of pandemic H1N1 influenza viruses in mice. *J Virol.*, 2010, 84, 8607–16.

[11] Houng, H-SH; Garner, J; Zhou, Y; Lyons, A; Kuschner, R; Deye, G; et al. Emergent 2009 influenza A(H1N1) viruses containing HA D222N mutation associated with severe clinical outcomes in the Americas. *J Clin Virol.*, 2012, 53, 12–5.

[12] Rykkvin, R; Kilander, A. Within-patient emergence of the Influenza A (H1N1)pdm09 HA1 222G variant and clear association with severe disease, Norway. *Eurosurveill.*, 2013, 18, 1–11.

[13] Ikonen, N; Haanpää, M; Rönkkö, E; Lyytikäinen, O; Kuusi, M; Ruutu, P; et al. Genetic diversity of the 2009 pandemic influenza A(H1N1) viruses in Finland. *PLoS One.*, 2010, 5, e13329.

[14] Miller, RR; MacLean, AR; Gunson, RN; Carman WF. Occurrence of haemagglutinin mutation D222G in pandemic influenza A(H1N1) infected patients in the West of Scotland, United Kingdom, 2009-10. *Eurosurveill.*, 2010, 22, 15, 19534.

[15] Ledesma, J; Pozo, F; Pérez Ruiz, M; Navarro, JM; Piñeiro, L; Montes, M; et al. Substitutions in position 222 of haemagglutinin of pandemic influenza A (H1N1) 2009 viruses in Spain. *J Clin Virol.*, 2011, 51, 75–8.

[16] Antón, A; Marcos, MA; Martínez, MJ; Ramón, S; Martínez, A; Cardeñosa, N; et al. D225G mutation in the hemagglutinin protein found in 3 severe cases of 2009 pandemic influenza A (H1N1) in Spain. *Diagn Microbiol Infect.*, 2010, 67, 207–8.

[17] Malato, L; Llavador, V; Marmier, E; Youssef, J; Balick Weber, C; Rozé, H; et al. Pandemic influenza A(H1N1) 2009: molecular characterisation and

duration of viral shedding in intensive care patients in Bordeaux, south-west France, May 2009 to January 2010. *Eurosurveill.*, 2011, 16, 1–7.

[18] Baldanti, F; Zanetti, A. Letter to the editor. Virological analysis of fatal influenza cases in the United Kingdom during the early wave of influenza in winter 2010/11. *Eurosurveill.*, 2011, 15, 2009–10.

[19] Puzelli, S; Facchini, M; Spagnolo, D; De Marco, MA; Calzoletti, L; Zanetti A; et al. Transmission of Hemagglutinin D222G Mutant Strain of Pandemic (H1N1) 2009 Virus. *Emerg Infect Dis.*, 2010, 16, 863–5.

[20] Puzelli, S; Facchini, M; De Marco, MA; Palmieri, A; Spagnolo, D; Boros, S; et al. Molecular surveillance of pandemic influenza A(H1N1) viruses circulating in Italy from May 2009 to February 2010: association between haemagglutinin mutations and clinical outcome. *Eurosurveill.*, 2010, 15, 3–5.

[21] Ruggiero, T; De Rosa, F; Cerutti, F; Pagani, N; Allice, T; Stella, ML; et al. A(H1N1)pdm09 hemagglutinin D222G and D222N variants are frequently harbored by patients requiring extracorporeal membrane oxygenation and advanced respiratory assistance for severe A(H1N1)pdm09 infection. *Influenza Other Respir Viruses.*, 2013, 7, 1416–26.

[22] Selleri, M; Piralla, A; Rozera, G; Giombini, E; Bartolini, B; Abbate, I; et al. Detection of haemagglutinin D222 polymorphisms in influenza A(H1N1)pdm09-infected patients by ultra-deep pyrosequencing. *Clin Microbiol Infect.*, 2013, 19, 668–73.

[23] Melidou, A; Gioula, G; Exindari, M; Chatzidimitriou, D; Diza, E; Malisiovas N. Molecular and phylogenetic analysis of the haemagglutinin gene of pandemic influenza H1N1 2009 viruses associated with severe and fatal infections. *Virus Res.*, 2010, 151, 192–9.

[24] Moussi, AE; Kacem, MABH; Pozo, F; Ledesma, J; Cuevas, MT; Casas, I; et al. Frequency of D222G haemagglutinin mutant of pandemic (H1N1) pdm09 influenza virus in Tunisia between 2009 and 2011. *Diagnostic Pathology.*, 2013, 8, 124.

[25] Wu, C; Cheng, X; Wang, X; Lv, X; Yang, F; Liu, T; et al. Clinical and molecular characteristics of the 2009 pandemic influenza H1N1 infection with severe or fatal disease from 2009 to 2011 in Shenzhen, China. *J Med Virol.*, 2013, 85, 405–12.

[26] DeVries, A; Wotton, J; Lees, C; Boxrud, D; Uyeki, T; Lynfield R. Neuraminidase H275Y and hemagglutinin D222G mutations in a fatal case of 2009 pandemic influenza A (H1N1) virus infection. *Influenza Other Respir Viruses.*, 2012, 6, e85–8.

[27] Vazquez-Perez, JA; Isa, P; Kobasa, D; Ormsby, CE; Ramírez-Gonzalez, JE; Romero-Rodríguez, DP; et al. A (H1N1) pdm09 HA D222 variants associated with severity and mortality in patients during a second wave in Mexico. *Virol J.*, 2013, 10, 41.

[28] Chan, PKS; Lee, N; Joynt, GM; Choi, KW; Cheung, JLK; Yeung, ACM; et al. Clinical and virological course of infection with haemagglutinin D222G mutant strain of 2009 pandemic influenza A (H1N1) virus. *J Clin Virol.*, 2011, 50, 320–4.

[29] Chen, H; Wen, X; To, KKW; Wang, P; Tse, H; Chan, JFW; et al. Quasispecies of the D225G substitution in the hemagglutinin of pandemic influenza A(H1N1) 2009 virus from patients with severe disease in Hong Kong, China. *J Infect Dis.*, 2010, 201, 1517–21.

[30] Mak, GC; Au, KW; Tai, LS; Chuang, KC; Cheng, KC; Shiu, TC; et al. Association of D222G substitution in haemagglutinin of 2009 pandemic influenza A (H1N1) with severe disease. *Eurosurveill.*, 2010, 15, 2009–10.

[31] Potdar, VA; Chadha, MS; Jadhav, SM; Mullick, J; Cherian, SS; Mishra AC. Genetic characterization of the influenza A pandemic (H1N1) 2009 virus isolates from India. *PLoS One.*, 2010, 5, e9693.

[32] Wang, B; Dwyer, DE; Soedjono, M; Shi, H; Matlho, K; Ratnamohan, M; et al. Evidence of the circulation of pandemic influenza (H1N1) 2009 with D222D/G/N/S hemagglutinin polymorphisms during the first wave of the 2009 influenza pandemic. *J Clin Virol.*, 2011, 52, 304–6.

[33] Nakajima, N; Sato, Y; Katano, H; Hasegawa, H; Kumasaka, T; Hata, S; Tanaka, S; Amano, T; Kasai, T; Chong, JM; Iizuka, T; Nakazato, I; Hino, Y; Hamamatsu, A; Horiguchi, H; Tanaka, T; Hasegawa, A; Kanaya, Y; Oku, R; Oya, T ST. Histopathological and immunohistochemical findings of 20 autopsy cases with 2009 H1N1 virus infection. *Mod Pathol.*, 2010, 25, 1–13.

[34] World Health Organization. *Clinical management of human infection with pandemic (H1N1)* 2009: revised guidance. Avaible http//www.who.int/int/crs/resourses/pubblications/swineflu/clinical_managment/en/index.html accessed 2012 Jun 25., 2009.

[35] Zarychanski, R; Stuart, TL; Kumar, A; Doucette, S; Elliott, L; Kettner, J; et al. Correlates of severe disease in patients with 2009 pandemic influenza (H1N1) virus infection. *CMAJ.*, 2010, 182, 257–64.

[36] Moher, D; Liberati, A; Tetzlaff, J; Altman, DG. Preferred reporting items for systematic reviews and meta-analyses: the PRISMA statement. *BMJ.*, 2009, 339 (b2535).

[37] Alonso, M; Rodríguez-Sánchez, B; Giannella, M; Catalán, P; Gayoso, J; López, Bernaldo; de Quirós, JC; et al. Resistance and virulence mutations in patients with persistent infection by pandemic 2009 A/H1N1 influenza. *J Clin Virol.*, 2011, 50, 114–8.

[38] Baldanti, F; Campanini, G; Piralla, A; Rovida, F; Braschi, A; Mojoli, F; et al. Severe outcome of influenza A/H1N1/09v infection associated with 222G/N polymorphisms in the haemagglutinin: a multicentre study. *Clin Microbiol Infect.*, 2011, 17, 1166–9.

[39] Valli, MB; Meschi, S; Selleri, M; Zaccaro, P; Ippolito, G; Capobianchi, MR. Evolutionary pattern of pandemic influenza (H1N1) 2009 virus in the late phases of the 2009 pandemic. *PLoSCurr.*, 2010, 2(RRN1149).

[40] Falcone, V; Bierbaum, S; Kern, W; Kontny, U; Bertz, H; Huzly, D; et al. Influenza virus A(H1N1)pdm09 hemagglutinin polymorphism and associated disease in southern Germany during the 2010/11 influenza season. *Arch Virol.*, 2013, 158, 1297–303.

[41] Zehender, G; Pariani, E; Piralla, A; Lai, A; Gabanelli, E; Ranghiero, A; et al. Reconstruction of the Evolutionary Dynamics of the A(H1N1)pdm09 Influenza Virus in Italy during the Pandemic and Post-Pandemic Phases. Guan Y. *PLoS One.*, 2012, 7, e47517.

[42] Valli, MB; Selleri, M; Meschi, S; Zaccaro, P; Vincenti, D; Lalle, E; et al. Hemagglutinin 222 Variants in Pandemic (H1N1) 2009 Virus. *Emerg Infect Dis.*, 2011, 17, 749–51.

[43] El Moussi, A; Pozo, F; Ben Hadj Kacem, MA; Ledesma, J; Cuevas, MT; Casas, I; et al. Virological Surveillance of Influenza Viruses during the 2008-09, 2009-10 and 2010-11 Seasons in Tunisia. *PLoS One.*, 2013, 8, e74064

In: Influenza and RNA Viruses
Editor: R. H. Bishop, pp. 25-54

ISBN: 978-1-63321-799-7

Chapter 2

NEW CANCER SYSTEMATIZATION: HYPOTHESIS OF THE CARCINOGENIC HYPERCYCLE

V. N. Malzev*

Urologisch-Onkologischer Arbeitskreis (UOA) Niedersachsen, Germany
Urologengenossenschaft Hannover (UroH), Germany

Abstract

To grasp the scientific information about cancer, its systematization is required. This systematization is conducted in the following succession, from general to particular: general theory of systems, theory of dissipative systems (synergetics), theory of life genesis based on hypercycles, and molecular biology.

In the context of such systematization, the process of cancerogenesis is scrutinized. Cancerogenesis is a process of continuous modification of gene expression in a cancerous cell due to epigenomic DNA methylation. The base of this process is one of the autocatalytic reactions as the simplest primary life form capable of replication, modification of species due to mutations, involving RNA reproduction of other cyclic reactions in the process, and competition with other replicative units. Such a reaction is

*E-mail addresses: wladimirm@web.de, wladimirmalzev@mail.ru

referred to as hypercycle. On the one hand, this hypercycle ensures self-reproduction, on the other hand, epigenetic DNA reprogramming, which entails cancerous cell transformation. A hypercycle capable of such reprogramming is referred to as cancerogenic hypercycle.

A cancerogenic hypercycle is generated at the beginning as an autonomous process of RNA replication in the cell cytoplasm which has stopped the cooperation with DNA replication. Under the impact of diverse factors, it obtains the ability of concurring with the DNA replication, becomes the new organizer of order in the cell and, by and by, displaces and depresses the latter one (DNA replication). The condition for generation of a cancerogenic hypercycle is a hypercyclic link of two and more cyclic reactions based on common ferments and (or) on a RNA interference mechanism.

The generation of a cancerogenic hypercycle is also regarded as the generation of a new regressive dissipative system and the associated possibility of mathematical modelling and prognosticating of this process.

In the article, possible structures and forms of cancerogenic hypercycles are mentioned, the cancerous hyper-cycle based on interaction between RdRP and dsRNA resulting from this as a revision of the anti-tumour impact of the radiation and chemotherapy is scrutinized, as well as new possibilities of cancer diagnostic and treatment.

The difference concerning the approach to cancer treatment between the modern target therapy conception and the proposed conception is shown.

PACS 87.17.-d, 87.16.-b, 87.16.-v

Keywords: Cancer, carcinogenic hypercycle, hypothesis of the carcinogenic hypercycle

1. Introduction. New Cancer Systematization

1.1. Choose of Knowledge System to Understand Cancer Nature

Any field of human activity without exception requires a certain knowledge organization. Organization means creation of a knowledge system in one or another field. Whereupon, the more complex and the more diverse this field is, the more important is it to organize it rightly. This concerns the field of scientific knowledge in general as well as the field of cancer studies in particular.

At the present, the number of factors concerning cancer studies has reached such a size, and their quality requires such specialized knowledge for their understanding that the leading of the sum of these diverse and numerous facts in an integral system is an insistent necessity. Modern existing cancer systematization based on histological, genetic and histochemical criteria is not sufficient to understand cancer nature; if the opposite would be the case, we would have found an effective way of cancer treatment. If we cannot treat cancer, this means we do not understand what it is, and if we do not understand what it is, this means we have systemized our knowledge wrongly.

The situation of knowledge flow reminds of the situation of a picture consisting of a number of pixels. We have divided the picture into lots of small elements-pixels with the hope to understand its deep sense, but as result, we have lost the understanding of the picture itself. If we by and by reduce the image resolution, certain fragments capable of being differentiated appear, from which a general picture can be composed, as we do when composing a puzzle. Having composed this puzzle, we will also understand the sense of its separate pixels.

This metaphor is to be treated with caution, understanding its narrowness, yet it transfers the sense of new systematization rightly, and this sense is concluded in the fact that the nature of what takes place in a cancerous cell should be tried to understand through larger fragments allowing to create an integral unitary picture and not scattered "pixels" in the form of molecules and biochemical reactions taking place between them, what we have at the present in oncology. These large fragments can be imagined in the form of separate processes taking place in a cancerous cell and mutually linked with each other. If we can extract these large fragments, we can understand their interaction with each other by their comparison in different biological species and at different evolution stages, and, as result, understand which processes entail cancer.

A disadvantage of the modern traditional systematization is also the fact that it takes chains of biochemical reactions for the base, which are regarded as predetermined. For example, there is such a term as "signal paths" "growth signals", on which the transformation of a normal cell to a cancerous one takes place [1]. That is, a direct cause and effect link is taken as the base, but the questions why this link has emerged and why it is of coincidental, statistic nature, are not scrutinized. Besides, self-sufficiency in growth signals is scrutinized, but no explanation is given to what exactly ensures such self-sufficiency. Like this, other specific features of a cancerous transformation are scrutinized: insensitivity to growth-inhibitory (antigrowth) signals, evasion of programmed cell death (apoptosis), limitless replicative potential, sustained angiogenesis, and tissue invasion and metastasis. That is, a description but no explanation of the cancerous transformation process is given.

Cancerous transformation is not a predetermined process. This is a probabilistic process. This is why for its understanding also probabilistic processes taking place in the living nature must be taken for the base. Before doing so, we must turn to the general theory of systems which deals with questions of knowledge systematization. We are not going to discuss this theory; we just point shortly at the very basic dispositions and rules according to which knowledge systematization is done and which directly concern our hypothesis.

According to the general theory of systems, any system consists of single parts elements. Choose of elements can also be arbitrary, but it has to be fulfilled according to a certain rule: only those system parts can be elements to which certain homogeneity is innate [2].

Separate elements become a system in the case where they are merged by a certain system-creating factor (Fig. 1). Such factors include, for example, repercussions [3]. It must be noted that in the scheme, only two elements are pointed out, for simplification. In reality, they can be multiple. According to

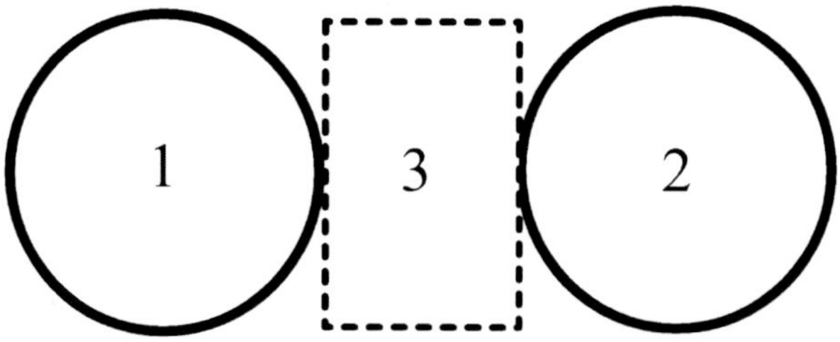

Figure 1. Separate elements 1 and 2 and uniting them in system a backbone factor 3.

the "monocentrism principle", a stable system is characterized by one center. If there is more than one of such centers, such system is characterized by instability, perturbation of coordination processes and de-organization. Such effects emerge when ones processes are laid onto other ones [4].

For hierarchical systems, the "law of hierarchical compensations" is typical which fixes the fact that "the real growth of diversity on the highest level is ensured by its effective inhibition on precedent levels" [5]. From this it follows that "growth of diversity at the lowest hierarchical level destroys the highest organization level" [6] and that "lack of inhibitions... entails destructuralization of the system as a whole" [5]. Any system is scrutinized within certain boundaries. This also concerns the knowledge system: we have to limit its application field from the beginning on.

1.2. Construction of a Normal Eukaryotic Cell Based on Replicatve Processes Running in It

So, bearing in mind the rules listed above, let us try to construct our cancer knowledge system in a new way. Let us begin with the last one, the narrowness of the knowledge field. In this given concrete case, we limit the cancer knowledge field by just knowledge about the cancerous cell only. We deliberately simplify the situation, not reckoning such information about cancer as e. g., organism immunity.

The second step is the choice of system elements based on certain criteria. Such a criterion, let us remind, is the relative homogeneity of the chosen elements. For this, we have to determine how a cancerous cell differs from a normal one and what they have in common. They have in common the fact that they are both replicative units in both cases DNA replication takes place. The difference between them is, firstly, the fact that a cancerous cell is a cell with a high level of mutations taking place in it, secondly, that a cancerous cell is regarded by some authors as a new life species [7] and thirdly, that a cancerous cell as a new life species is more primitive in its construction in comparison to a normal cell.

Assuming this, we have to find cell system elements which would correspond to these listed features.Such elements we already have mentioned this particularity must be large enough for us to be able to compose our "puzzle" from them. We find these elements which correspond to all listed criteria in the theory of life genesis based on hypercycles M. Eigen, P. Schuster "The Hypercycle. A Principle of Nature Self-Organization" [8]. The principle of the replication of DNA and RNA as separate elements with different mutation levels was laid in the basis of this theory. Thereby, RNA replication is a more primitive life form than DNA replication, and life evolution is presented as development from RNA replication to DNA replication, whereupon hypercycles are the mechanism of such development. The feature of homogeneity of such elements is the replication ability, and the distinctive feature is the different mutagenicity levels.

Moreover, we also add the theory of life genesis based on ribozymes which has not entered the theory of hypercycles. Its base is the principle of RNA self-replication where it plays the role of genetic information carrier as well as of the replication catalyst. Ribozyme replication also can be placed in the line of elements as corresponding to the features listed above: replication and mutagenicity.

1.3. RNA and DNA Worlds. Description of Their Interaction in Prokaryotes and Eukaryotes

Therefore, we can highlight two system elements: DNA replication (which we in the future refer to as "DNA world") and RNA replication (which is in the future referred to as "RNA world").

These two elements are merged in a system in the way that the RNA world is a component of the DNA world and is in hierarchical subordination to it. Such a designation is appropriate also from the evolutional point of view because the RNA world, according to the theory of life development, is a predecessor of the modern DNA world. The nature of the relationship of the DNA and RNA worlds differs in different species. If virus reproduction in the cell takes place with a high mutagenicity level and emerging of new virus strains, the bacterial cell mutates not that often, and a highly differentiated cell of a multiple-cell organism does not mutate at all, and if it does, it becomes a cancerous cell. Such difference in mutations frequency is obviously explained by different hierarchical mechanisms between the DNA and the RNA world. If we take the cardinal situation, on one of its poles such hierarchy lacks completely, which can be observed e. g., in virus reproduction in the cell, and in the other one, in highly differentiable organism cells, it is developed most strongly. The nature of the hierarchical interaction of the DNA and RNA worlds in a bacterial cell lies in the middle, between these two poles.

We therefore see that for a highly developed life species standing on a higher evolutional level, the lack ob mutability is distinctive. In this sense, cancer is a more primitive life form in comparison to multiple-cell organisms.

If we search for differences between a bacterial cell and a highly differentiated organism cell according to the criterion of hierarchy of the RNA and DNA worlds, we realize that it consists of the existence of nucleus membrane in an eukaryotoc highly differentiated cell and the lack of such membrane in a prokaryotic bacterial cell.

According to the general system theory, DNA and RNA worlds correspond on Fig. 1 with the elements marked by nrs. 1 and 2, and the system-creating factor marked by nr. 3 and merging these elements into a unitary system of a normal differentiated cell, is the existence of a nucleus membrane. This system-creating factor is of hierarchical nature: RNA world is inferior to the DNA world.

The hierarchical regulation is realized by a certain structure of the nucleus membrane the pore complex which plays the role of the dispatcher who regulates the flows of chemical substances between the nucleus and the cytoplasm. Naturally, such hierarchical regulation is not limited by the pore complex only. Other factors also are also concerned with such regulation.For example, they contain the repression of ferment synthesis when switching off of the correspondent genes takes place, translating repression which runs with emergence of masked mRNA, total regulation (regulation by means of phosphokinase [9]). Recently, also control by means of micro RNA has been counted to such regulation [10].

Limiting the system-creating factor by the pore complex only, we deliberately simplify the situation to understand the difference of the interactions between the DNA and RNA world in prokaryotes and eukaryotes.

The impact of the system-creating factor in the form of a pore complex of the nucleus membrane disappears either during the mitosis period when the cell membrane itself disappears or at the cost of affection of the pore complex itself which takes place during cancerous cell transformation. For a cancerous tumour, generation of pathological forms and prolonging of the mitosis metaphase is characteristic [11].Affection of the pore complex during cancerous cell transformation is also already proven [12]. This question is discussed more concretely below.

In both cases, the RNA world gains a possibility of separating and self-organization.

1.4. Cyclic Processes as Elements of a Dissipative System

Any life form is not just a system, but a dissipative system [13]. A separate eukaryotic cell is not an exception from this rule. As it is mentioned by Rysnichenko G. Yu.,

> "From the point of view of the dynamic systems theory, a cell is a dissipative structure. According to the determination of I. R. Prygozhin, a dissipative structure is an open system which keeps itself

> in a thermodynamically imbalanced but structurally stable state at the cost of flows of material and energy. The terminus dissipative stresses the fact that keeping the structure requires energy input (dissipation).
>
> A specific feature of dissipative structures is the ability to spontaneous emergence of new order forms. If the energy flow increases, the system can come to a point of instability called bifurcation point after the passing of which the system can run a very different way which would allow emergence of new structures and ordered forms[1] ." [14]

Dissipative systems were firstly explored in a lifeless world, which speaks in favour of their natural universality. The volume of the given article allows us to describe separate features of a dissipative system only very generally and compactly. Such feature include:

1. Self-organization from chaos by Thom catastrophe and the bifurcation point.
2. Opening of the system. Needness of continiuous energy flow.
3. Imbalance of the system, i. e., perturbation of balance between its elements.
4. Spontaneity of emergence and probability linked with it (and not predetermination) of emergence of a new dissipative system.
5. Non-lined nature of processes running in it.
6. Sensitivity to original conditions.
7. Irreversibility of running processes, "once and for all"-principle.

If we regard the cell as a dissipative system, the cell cycle also is logically to be regarded as a period of time from the emerging of such system to the termination of its existence. The point of existence beginning and the point of existence termination is the bifurcation point in which, by Thom catastrophe, coincidentally a new dissipative system is formed. So, every cell division corresponds to deintegration of the dissipative system up to component elements DNA and RNA

[1] authors translation

worlds, and creation of two new dissipative systems: stem and daughter cells, based on these deintegrated elements by Thom catastrophe mentioned above.

During the existence period of a dissipative system the interphase period the DNA world is superior over the RNA world at the cost of the evolutional advantage in the form of regulation by the nuclear pore complex. During the deintegration and existence termination period of the dissipative system the mitosis period two new dissipative systems are formed where different RNA worlds changed before by DNA worlds at the cost of DNA methylation re-code differently the DNA of new created cells. At the moment of cell division, the probability of DNA world superiority over the RNA world, i. e., emergence of a normal system-creating factor, is higher than the probability of a different system organization. As a result of the perturbed interaction of these worlds, reasons of which are discussed below, the probability of this different system organization increases significantly. According to our hypothesis, this different system organization is a cancerogenic hypercyle which we discuss below.

In case of the real emergence of such self-organization we speak of the beginning of cancerogenesis, i. e., of emergence of a mutant clone of cancer cells. Original conditions, to which a dissipative system is sensitive here the nature of DNA methylation determine to a significant extent the nature of the cancerogenesis itself: tumor growth speed, its invasiveness, and ability to metastasize.

Besides the mentioned dissipative system features, other features are also innate to a cancerogenesis, such as irreversibility of running processes and their non-lined nature. The latter feature means that insignificant changes of one parameter of the dissipative system, e.g., of the RNA world enzyme, entails quite significant changes of its another parameter, e. g., of the DNA world enzyme.

1.5. RNA and DNA Worlds. Describing Their Interaction with Each Other in a Normal Cell

The DNA world differs from the RNA world by the existence of a double spiral in the DNA, a re-combination apparatus for correcting the replication mistakes. At the cost of the existence of this double spiral and the re-combination of DNA areas, the number of mistakes during the replication is

$$1 \cdot 10^{-9} \tag{1}$$

There is a different situation during the RNA replication [8]. In the case of RNA replication, the number of mistakes is

$$1 \cdot 10^{-4} \tag{2}$$

In this way, RNA replication is a much more mutagenic process than DNA replication. In fact, viral RNA replication very often entails generation of new viruses. Examples for such mutations are emergence of the poultry plague virus, the swine influenza virus. And the virus of common influenza is also subject to frequent mutations.

Generally, viruses are one of the expressions of the RNA world, and their self-organization is of a diverse nature. They can accrete and destroy the cell, their genetic apparatus can enter the genetic apparatus of the cell, and, according to our hypothesis, they can participate in creation of a cancerogenic hypercycle, which is discussed below.

The next already mentioned difference of the RNA world from the DNA world is the fact that the RNA world, being a consisting part of the DNA world, is also capable of autonomous development. RNA is able to replicate also without participation of DNA. Such process can take place with participation of cytoplasm replicases as well as at the cost of the RNA itself which possesses catalyzing activity. It is important to mention here that the RNA world in the boundaries of the cell can exist autonomously, without participation of the DNA, but the DNA world cannot exist without the RNA world. DNA cannot produce protein which is necessary for its own replication directly, without participation of matrix RNA and transport RNA.

The third difference between the RNA and the DNA world is the different position in relation to energetic cell resources. The RNA world is positioned closer to these resources than the DNA world. Before entering the cell nucleus, the ATP enters the RNA world from mitochondria.

The fourth difference or, more precisely, speciality of the DNA world which makes it different from the RNA world is the already mentioned earlier existence of a semi-permeable nucleus envelope which accomplishes the function of cooperation of the DNA and RNA worlds and ensures their hierarchy. We have referred the existence of the cell membrane to the DNA world because without it, existence of a RNA world is possible, but existence of a DNA world in eukaryotes is impossible.

2. An Abstract Cancerogenic Hypercycle

2.1. Construction of a Cancerous Eukaryotic Cell Based on Replicative Processes Running in It

According to the Eigen and Schuster theory of life genesis, life was generated and developed originally as a competition of hypercycles.

A hypercycle is a method of merging self-reproducing macromolecules to closed autocatalytic chemical cycles. A hypercycle is several cyclical reactions which are organized in a way in which by-products of one reaction are catalysts of another one, and the last reaction products a catalyst for the first one. This is a mean of merging self-reproducing units to a new, enduring system which is capable of evolution. [8].

Darwins selection which is a pre-condition for emergence of hypercycles can, on a molecular level, have a place in systems which have features for metabolism, self-reproduction and, which is important for the suggested hypothesis, mutability. The latter one always accompanies self-reproduction.

The predecessor of a hypercycle is a common cycle, called differently self-replicating unit or strengthened auto-catalyst. An example of such self-replicating unit is multiplication of a RNA-containing phage in a bacterial cell. RNA, using the translation apparatus of the host cell, entails emergence of a protein which, in its turn, contributes to multiplication of infectious RNA.

A hypercycle consists of mutually linked cycles. Taking the precedent example of multiplication of phage RNA and presuming that the protein synthesized with its participation will also have features of a catalyst of any other process which, in its turn, will catalyze the emergence of phage RNA in the cell, we will already get a hypercycle.

According to the Eigen and Schuster theory, hypercycles of such kind have detached from each other in separate compartments, i.e., certain boxes of the cell where certain biochemical reactions run, after what they have become simple replicating units. Examples for such compartments are the cell nucleus where DNA replication takes place, or ribosome where translation takes place. An example for a simple replication unit is DNA replication in the nucleus and replication of virus RNA in the cytoplasm [8].

It is known from synergetic that different genera can avoid competition if they occupy different ecological niches [15]. The competition principle does not only apply to biological genera, but also to systems of molecular level [8].

Similar processes take place in the cell, where DNA replication in the nucleus and RNA replication in the cytoplasm play the role of competing genera, earlier designated by us as DNA world and RNA world.

In the process of evolution, at the cost of isolation of these processes from each other by means of the nuclear membrane, the competition has stopped and was replaced by cooperation. In Fig. 2, these worlds and their interaction with each other at different stages of cell transformation are presented. As we

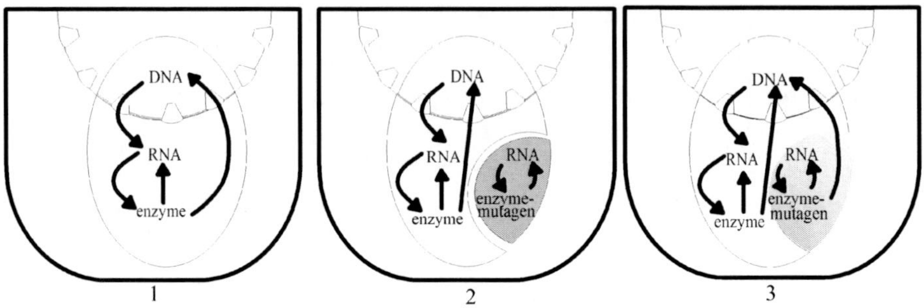

Figure 2. Co-activation of the DNA world and the RNA world (grey) at different levels of development of the carcinogenic cell transformation
1 - DNA world in a normal cell, 2 - Autonomy and generation of the RNA world, 3 - Development of the RNA world. Under special conditions (see text), carcinogenic hyper-cycle is developed (RNA world) which grasps for the DNA world, so that the courses of the DNA world are included to it.

see, for DNA replication a translation apparatus is required which belongs to the RNA world. Thus, the RNA world is an integral part of the DNA world, but nevertheless it is capable of autonomous functioning. It must be said that by RNA world, we understand not only the replication of the viral RNA with use of the host cell resources, but also the whole translation apparatus with participation of the matrix RNA as well as of the transport RNA, as well as the ribozym. In the presented hypothesis we limit ourselves to the description of one of the possible forms of the RNA world, the cancerogenic hypercycle which entails cancerogenic cell transformation.

A viral RNA, a matrix RNA, a transport RNA or a masked matrix RNA can be a RNA source for such hypercycle in the cell. For the suggested hypothesis, it is unimportant from which RNA exactly the carcinogenic hypercycle is formed, which is described further, but it is important that any RNA capable of translation is able to form a cancerogenic hypercycle as well.

So, according to the general theory of systems, DNA and RNA worlds correspond on Fig. 1 to the elements designed by 1 and 2, and the system-creating factor designed by nr. 3 and merging these elements into a system of a cancerous eukaryotic cell, is the hypercyclic link. This hypercyclic link is the interaction factor of the RNA world with the DNA world. As a system-creating factor, this hypercyclic link replaces the system-creating factor of a normal cell in the form of a pore complex of the nuclear membrane. How exactly emerges and develops this hypercyclic link is shown by us below.

2.2. Mechanism of Acting of Cancerogenic Factors in the Light of the Proposed Hypothesis. Strengthening Factors of a Separate Cyclic Replicative Reaction

Examining the mechanism of the impact of canerogenic factors on the cell, we have to take in consideration not only the impact of these factors on concrete chemical substances, but, even more, also their impact on concrete worlds described. All cancerogens entail perturbation of the balance between the DNA and the RNA world in favor of the RNA world in the case of emergence of a state of competition between them. They are therefore able to ensure the selective advantage of the RNA world in relation to the DNA world in the case of emergence of such state.

1. Impact of radioactive radiation of the DNA and the RNA world entails different consequences. In the DNA world, mutations caused by DNA damage entail strengthening of reparation processes of the damaged areas, which requires additional energy consumption. In the RNA world, radiation will cause strengthened mutations generation, strengthened mutagenesis without any following participation of reparation processes. No additional energy consumption takes place due, as a general rule, to absence of reparation processes in the RNA world. A part of the energy produced by the cell is therefore spent on restoration of the DNA world, which entails reduction of resources which are required for control of the RNA world. Thus, as a more highly organized structure, the DNA world suffers from radiation more than the RNA world. Such innovating mechanism, however, is functioning with a weak radiation when as a result of its impact, the number of mutations in the RNA world does not rise above a certain number, about

$$1 \cdot 10^{-4} \quad (3)$$

If the intensity of the radiation entails a higher number of mutations, not only DNA is killed, but also the RNA world, and the cell stops its existence. Obviously, by this mechanism is explained, amongst others, in line with deceleration of cell division, the healing effect of radiation therapy and induction of tumors by weak but continuous radiation.

2. Chemical cancerogens act by the same principle, with the only difference that certain chemical cancerogens cause certain mutations, which probably become a consisting part of the cancerogenic hypercycle.

3. Viruses cause strengthening of the RNA world at the cost of their own replication. Actually, they are an autonomous RNA world themselves with their entering into the cell cytoplasm. At the cost of their impact, the balance between the DNA and the RNA world in favor of the latter is perturbed in turn.

4. Loss of the DNA world control over the RNA world. A possible explanation for such loss can be ageing of the DNA world. The number of replications of the DNA world is finite in a normal cell. The limiting takes place at the cost of the loss of the DNA substance at each cell division [16]. A weakening of the DNA world as a result of its ageing entails automatic strengthening of the RNA world in the case of starting of a competing interaction with it.

5. Strengthening of the RNA world at the cost of additional impact of DNA world enzymes on the RNA replication or mutual strengthening of two cyclic reactions.

   Interaction of cyclic replicative reactions in a hypercycle was discussed in the book M. Eigen, P. Schuster [8]. Basing on the analysis of such interaction, let us shortly take a look on the interaction of two cyclic reactions of DNA and RNA replication in a hypercycle (Fig. 3).

   On Fig. 3, two cyclic hypercycle elements are shown consisting correspondingly of a pair of DNA and RNA-directed DNA polymerase (DP) and a pair of gene-polymerase RNA and RNA polymerase (RP), and the mechanism of enhancement of the RNA replication in a hypercycle is shown as well. The condition for the emerging of such hypercycle is expression of genes which ensure the enzyme synthesis for RNA replication.

In the case where DP and RP more favor more RNA than DNA, the winner is RNA. This case is shown on Fig. 3. In the case where the links are equally strong, mutual strengthening of two cyclic reactions DNA replication and RNA replication takes place. Under DNA replication, not strengthening of the DNA world as a unitary hierarchical system is to be understood, but strengthening of the separately taken DNA replication itself, accompanied by uncontrolled cell division.

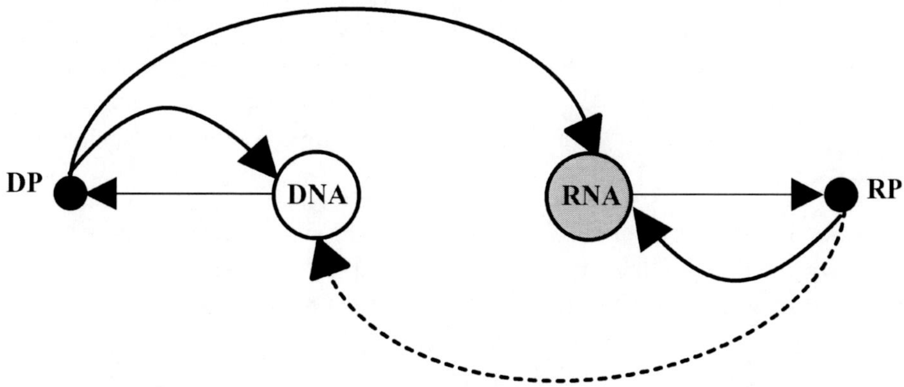

Figure 3. RNA replication strengthening as a result of competitive interaction with DNA replication in a hyper cycle.
DNA and RNA coding the own polymerases RNA-directed DNA polymerase (DP) and RNA polymerase (RP). If DP and RP more favor RNA than DNA, that becomes the winner RNA and DNA dies out.Continuous lines specify, what communications are preferable.

The number of such cyclic elements building the hypercycle can be more than two. In such case, the situation with an advantage of one or another cyclic element complicates. In this case, to rate the advantage of a separately taken cyclic element, appliance of a more complex mathematical apparatus and computer modelling is required.

2.3. Interaction of the DNA and RNA Worlds in a Malignant Cell

The essence of our hypothesis results in the fact that in a cell, a cancerogenic hypercycle of a special kind, the RNA world hypercycle, at the cost of the regained competition advantage, is able to develop independently and gradually displace the DNA world replication, which is inherent to a normally functioning cell (Fig. 2). We understand under a cancerogenic hypercycle one of the forms of development and expression of the RNA world in the cell. As a result of the causes described below, a simple replication unit, here the RNA world, gains the features of a hypercycle of second or higher level which starts to have competing interrelations with the replication unit the DNA world.

As it is mentioned by Eigen and Schuster,

> "The hypercycle is competing with any separated replication unit which does not belong to the hypercycle, independent of whether it is independent, a part of another hypercycle or even linked to the given hypercycle by a parasite bound. The hypercycle can grow or reduce its size if such a modification gives a selective advantage[2] ." [8].

So, besides one center in the system, an additional center emerges, and such system according to the "monocentrism principle" of the general theory of systems described above becomes instable, coordination processes are perturbed in it. According to another law of this theory, "law of hierarchical compensations", "growth of diversity at the bottom hierarchical level destroys the top level of the organization", i. e., unlimited RNA replication mutability destroys the DNA world system.

Evolutional regress takes place at the cell level.

If the RNA replication in a normal cell sometimes runs with a high mutability, which we can see in the case of viral RNA replication, it is quite right to presume that a similar process is possible not only in relation to viral RNA, as all necessary elements of such mutable replication are contained in a normal cell.

It must be stressed that examples of a similar replacing of the DNA by RNA exist in the nature. Highly organized organisms can be displaced by more simple ones. Biomolecules, under the impact of new life conditions, drop the part of genetic information without which they can not only get along now, but moreover get the possibility to reproduce faster we talk about RNA molecules of certain phages [15].

Thus, cancer can be regarded as a state of competition of two worlds, two replication processes, which has changed the state of their cooperation. This is

[2] authors translation

an organization of a new order by means of cancelling the old one. As a result of this new competition and the chaos developed in the cell, the RNA world becomes the new organizer of the order, replacing the precedent organizer of the order the DNA world.

At the very beginning of the cancerogenesis, isolation takes place, autonomization of the simple reproductive RNA unit at the cost of the impact of the cancerogenic factors listed above. Here, the process can stop, what actually takes place in a common viral affection (see Fig. 2, nr 1).

Here, the "law of hierarchical compensations" applies. According to this law Lack of limits... entails destructuralization of the system as a whole. This means, lacking control from the side of the DNA world what actually happens during RNA world autonomization system destructuralization can take place.

If, as a result of mutations which happen during RNA replication, an enzyme emerges, which not only has a function which ensures RNA replication, but also a function of the oligo-nucleotide mutagen described below, the process of cell transformation develops further. Thus, the cancerogenic hypercycle gains the nature of a hypercycle of first level, i.e., consists of two components, where protein replicates RNA at the cost of auto-catalyst on the one side and is capable of DNA modification on the other side, and the RNA is linked with it by means of cyclic feedback (see Fig. 2, nr. 2). In our case, the simplest cancerogenic hypercycle or the first level hypercycle produces a protein-enzyme which causes DNA modification by its methylation. Thus, the enzyme which accomplishes the role of the intermediator causes replication of mutant RNA on the one side and ensures continuous process of DNA modification on the other side.

A speciality of the cancerogenic hypercycle is the fact that it is not a hypercycle of second level in the strict, classical understanding of this word. In a classical second level hypercycle, the information medium, here the RNA, provides an instruction of two types. Firstly, for its own re-generation, secondly, for emergence of the second type ferment, here the protein-mutagen which changes either the cell DNA directly or indirectly by RNA mutations and emergence of new kinds of protein, which, in their turn, act as mutagens on DNA, perturbing acetylation and methylation of its oligo-nucleotides. But this is only one consisting part of the cancerogenic hypercycle, the original cancerogenic hypercycle (Fig. 4 nr. 1).

The classic hypercycle is two or more cyclic auto-catalyzing reactions where the reaction product of one cycle increases the reaction speed of the other cycle. In the cancerogenic hypercycle, however, in difference to the Eigen-Schuster hypercycle, the principle of strengthening of one cycle by the other one itself is kept, but instead of the product of a chemical reaction which strengthens the other cycle, changed structures and functions of the cancerous cell take place in such a role of strengthener (Fig. 4).

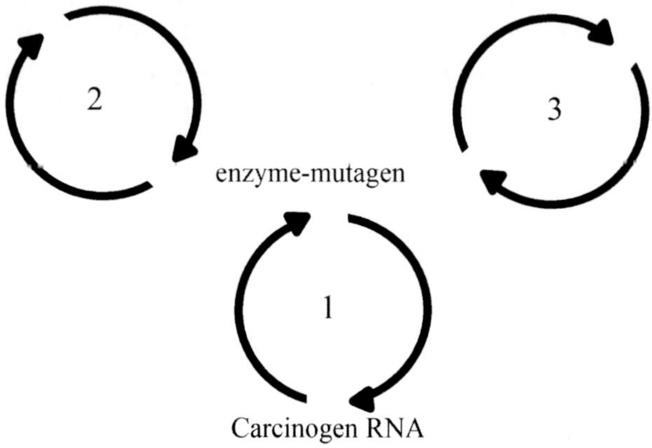

Figure 4. 1.Original carcinogenic hyper-cycle
2. Perturbation of the pore complex structure which enhances the original carcinogenic hyper-cycle
3. Unlimited cell division which enhances the carcinogenic hyper-cycle.

2.3.1. Change of the Cancerous Cell Structure

At the cost of the change of the pore complex structure and affection of transporter proteins of the RNA, Nup214 and Nup88 [12], loss of the RNA world control by the DNA world on the one side and weakening of the DNA world itself on the other side takes place.

For a cancerous tumour, generation of pathological forms and prolonging of the mitosis metaphase is distinctive [11]. This is why the time of absence of a cell membrane in the mitosis process in a cancerous cell increases in comparison to such time in a normal cell, and the forming of a cancerogenic hypercycle is facilitated.

Remember that DNA replication is only possible with participation of the RNA world which is separated from it by a pathologically changed pore complex. Loss of control of the translation entails automatically strengthening of the RNA world, uncontrolled RNA replication. This process is designated on Fig. 4 by nr. 2.

2.3.2. Change of the Cancerous Cell Function

Submission of the DNA world to the RNA world is expressed by the fact that the DNA world gains features of the RNA world: mutability and illimitability of replication. RNA replication can theoretically continue for an unlimited period of time in case of replication of a pathogenic virus. Practically, it is limited by resources of the cell. In the case of unlimited cancerous cell division, this limit is cancelled. The DNA world gets involved in supporting of the RNA world cycle at the cost of unlimited cancerous cell division.

As a result of DNA modifications described above, i. e., changes of the epigenomic code and re-programming of DNA, gene expression takes place which stimulates cell division.

This process is designated on Fig. 4 by nr. 3. The structure of a cancerogenic hypercycle can be different, but in any case it includes a cancerogenic RNA and an enzyme-mutagen which ensures widening of the RNA world at the cost of involving of the DNA world structures in it.

2.4. Distributing of Cell Resources as a Result of the Development of a Cancerogenic Hypercycle

As a result of the emergence and development of a cancerogenic hypercycle related to displacing and replacing of the DNA world by the RNA world, energetic cell resources in the form of ATP (adenosine triphosphate) begin to re-distribute in favor of the RNA world the more of these resources are gained by the RNA world, the less of them remain for the DNA world. The energetic cell resources are limited. They are especially limited in the case of a cancerous cell transformation when aerobic glycolysis is replaced by anaerobic glycolysis, and ATP production decreases by several times. For the DNA world to be able to keep the genetic information unchanged, continuous reparation of mutating genes is necessary, what is accomplished by ferments which repair the damaged mutating areas. These ferments are able to accomplish such work only if there is sufficient energy because DNA reparation processes are highly energy-consuming. This is why lack of a sufficient flow of energy in the form of ATP mutations begin which are not repaired; what is called genetic instability begins. Remember that the DNA world is a dissipative system, i.e., a system which can only exist with the condition of continuous energy flow. In the case of absence of such flow it dissociates as a system.

Besides energetic resources, resources of translation apparatus also redistribute in favor of the RNA world. The part of the translation apparatus which was busy supplying the DNA world, e. g., synthesis of the same enzymes for DNA reparation, cannot any longer supply the cell with such synthesis after being displaced by the RNA world. Instead, the translation apparatus changes to enzyme synthesis for the replication of the cancerogenic hypercycle. As a result, the DNA world loses the ability of self-restoration, and the RNA world, in opposite, progresses.

2.5. Mutual Relations of Epigenomic and Genetic Processes in a Cancerous Cell

Having begun as an epigenetic DNA modification process, a cancerogenic hypercycle entails at the end genetic perturbations in a cancerous cell. Scrutinizing epigenetic and genetic theories of cancer emergence, we simply watch different cancerogenesis stages which overlap each other, although they have a certain chronology: DNA modification first, then genetic DNA perturbations. The proposed hypothesis of the cancerogenic hypercycle cancels the contradiction between the epigenomic and the genetic theory of cancer emergence.

3. A Possible Real Cancerogenic Hypercycle

3.1. RNA Interference in a Normal Cell

A possible example of a cancerogenic hypercycle is modification of cell DNA by means of RNA interference mechanism. To understand the development mechanism of a cancerogenic hypercycle via RNA interference, it is necessary to stop shortly at how RNA interference functions in a normal cell.

Normally, the transcription and translation regulation runs the way pre-miRNA interaction with Dicer interaction with RISC. Hence, the "epigenetic code" of a normal cell is realized (Fig. 5). Pre-miRNA as well as dsRNA interact with the same structures in the cell cytoplasm with the protein complex Dicer and the RISC complex (RNA-induced silencing complex), whose central element is endonuclease which belongs to the proteins family Argonaute (Ago).

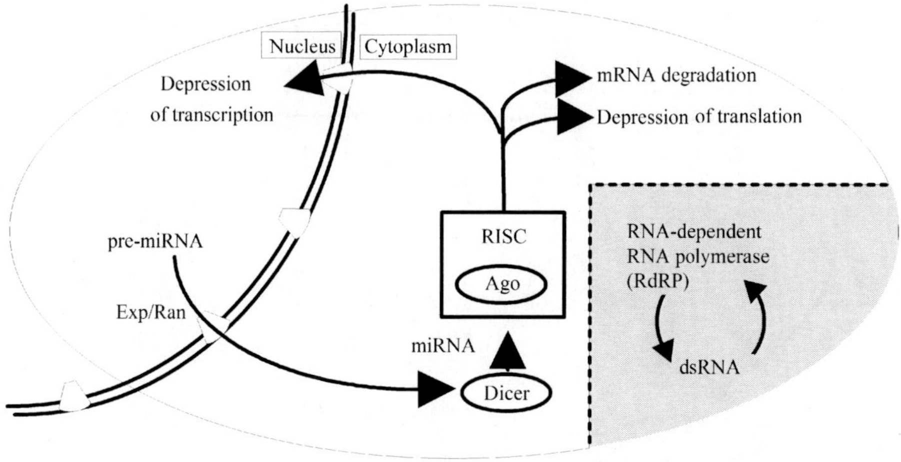

Figure 5. Transkription und translation regulation through RNA interference in a normal cell.Border between DNA world and RNA world (grey) is indicated by a dotted line.

These two classes of short RNAs, miRNA and siRNA, are able to compete for place in the same effectorial complexes [17], i.e., Dicer and RISC are the shared element which links two cyclic reactions: miRNA replication reaction and dsRNA replication reaction, and hence is a possible way of forming a hypercyclic link.

3.2. RNA Interference in a Cancer Cell

A cancerous hypercycle based on RNA interference is created in the following way (see Fig. 6). Two elements Dicer and RISC are a place of competing interaction between pre-miRNA and dsRNA where competing replacing of the miRNA regulating normally the gene transcription and translation by the cancerogenic dsRNA takes place. After such replacing, dsRNA becomes an antisense siRNA chain, the latter one methylates and modifies the DNA in the cell nucleus on the one hand, i. e., it modifies the normal "epigenetic code", and depresses the translation by binding it with the correspondent complementary sequence in the mRNA composition on the other hand.

siRNAs are capable of building up to long RNA molecules. Hence, they are able to be primers for synthesis of new RNAs on a single-stranded and / or a

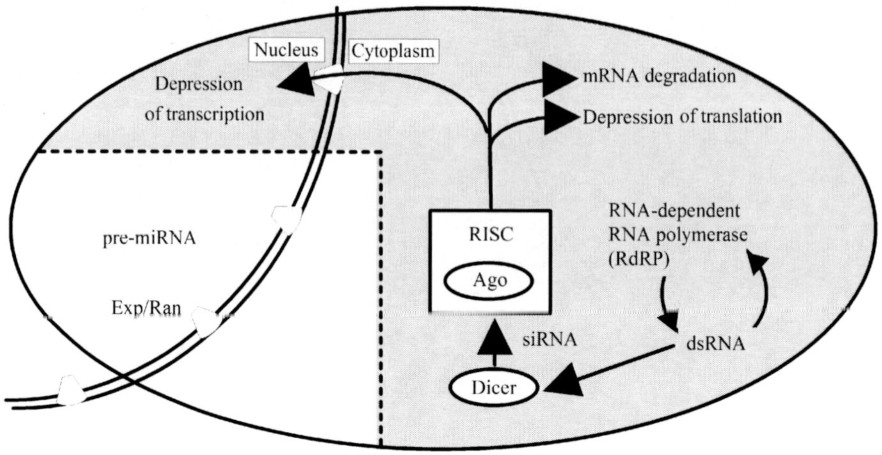

Figure 6. Spreading of the carcinogenic hypercycle (RdRP-dsRNA) on translation and transcription through RNA interference in a cancerous cell. Border between DNA world (left below) and RNA world (grey) is indicated by a dotted line.

double-stranded RNA matrix of the RNA-dependent RNA polymerase (RdRP) [18].

Prolonging siRNA products are double-stranded RNA themselves. This is why they are subject to further post-transcriptional modification with creation of "secondary" siRNAs and a probable participation of Dicer. Hence, the RNA interference process looks like a degrading polymerase chain reaction in which primary siRNA molecules, being primers for synthesis of new double-stranded RNA molecules, entail creation of secondary siRNAs.

This process can be autocatalytic, i. e., capable of autonomous evolution, and correspond to a hypercycle if one of the products of this cyclic reaction is emergence of ferments strengthening the cancerogenic hypercycle (discussed below).

Such cycle can continue indefinitely as long as a RNA is present which is able to be a matrix for siRNA primers [18].

Therefore, the cyclic reaction of *dsRNA - hypercycle strengthening ferments*, as a result of gaining a competing advantage over the cyclic translation *miRNA - mRNA degradation + Depression of translation* (see Fig. 5) control reaction, by the RNA interference mechanism displaces and replaces the latter one (see

Fig. 6). On a molecular level, this is expressed in decrease of miRNA concentration and increase of siRNA concentration.

3.3. Ferments Which Strenghten the Hypercycle. Strenghtening of the Cyclic Reaction as a Result of Different Enzyme Impact on Separate Hypercycle Elements

On Fig. 3 it was shown how the strengthening of the cyclic reaction of the RNA replication in an abstract cancerogenic hypercycle takes place. A similar strengthening can take place according to a similar scheme in case of a real cancerogenic hypercycle.

dsRNA can be a cyclic reaction which serves as the base for a cancerogenic hypercycle created by RNA interference (see Fig. 7, right area in the form of a circle of grey colour, limited by a dashed line) already described above, and any ferment able to cause RNA-dependent RNA replication can be the enzyme. Such an enzymatic activity is possessed by RNA-dependent RNA polymerase (RdRP) (see 2 Fig. 7), DNA-dependent RNA polymerase II (see 1 Fig. 7), retroviral reverse transcriptases reverse transcriptase (also known as revertase or RNA-directed DNA polymerase (see 3 Fig. 7) [18]. Presence of ferments able to catalyze different cyclic reactions is a typical feature of a hypercyclic link (see Fig. 3). The cyclic dsRNA replication reaction is supported by the enzyme RNA dependent RNA polymerase (RdRP) (see 2 Fig. 7). The strengthening of this reaction by other enzymes takes places in the following way. After the dsRNA becomes siRNA, the latter one (see 4 Fig. 7) modificates the DNA in such way that expression of genes of group A and group B takes place. Expression of genes of group A entails emergence of ferments which strengthen dsRNA replication. These ferments include e. g., DNA-dependent RNA polymerase II. Besides, in case of RNA virus replication, additional impact on the cyclic dsRNa replication reaction can be made by RNA directed DNA polymerase.

Expression of genes of group B entails to switching on of the mechanism of DNA replication and cell division.

In the case of a hypercycle with two cyclic reactions in our case, i. e., cyclic dsRNA replication reaction and mRNA replication the winner of the competition will be dsRNA, i. e., the RNA world, as RdRP replicates only dsRNA, but cannot replicate mRNA. Yet, the DNA-dependent RNA polymerase II can replicate mRNA as well as dsRNA. Hence, in sum, these two ferments

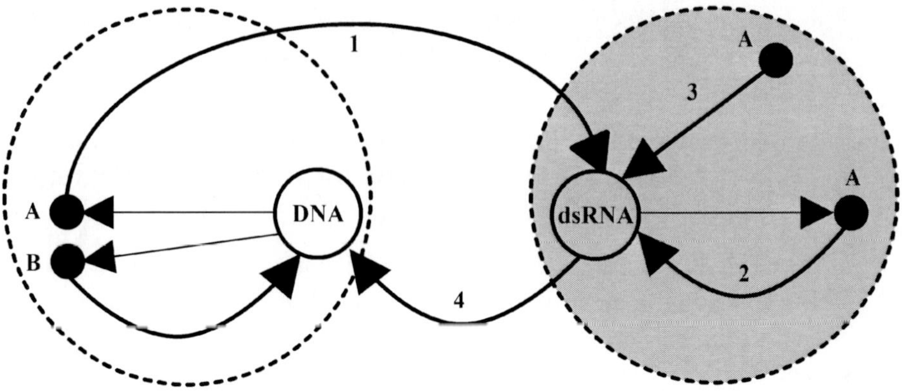

Figure 7. Competitive interaction of cyclic reactions of DNA -replication (circle dashed line at the left) and RNA-replication (circle of gray color on the right, limited to a dashed line) in a cancerogenic hyper cycle.
A - enzymes of replication of dsRNA
B - enzymes of replication of DNA and cellular division
1 - DNA-depend RNA polymerase II
2 - RNA-depend RNA polymerase (RdRP)
3 - RNA-directed DNA polymerase 4 - siRNA
(Explanations in the text).

more favor dsRNA than mRNA.

If a third cyclic reaction joins the hypercycle, in our case a revertase able to replicate dsRNA as well as a virus, the advantage of the RNA world even grows as a third ferment is added which strengthens dsRNA replication.

3.4. Falsifiability of the Proposed Hypothesis

In the case of the creation of a cancerous hypercycle by RNA interference, siRNA increase at the background of miRNA decrease takes place. Such profile speaks in favor of our hypothesis. Some facts confirming such development of incidents in a cancerous cell are already proven.Such facts include high dsRNA mutability and its capability of an autonomous replication, independently of the DNA world.

siRNA, as a dsRNA product, causes cancerogenic effect in a cell [19]. The capability of competition for the epigenetic regulation of transcription and translation between the siRNA of a cancerous hypercycle and the miRNA of the DNA world via the interference mechanism mentioned above in the section A possible real cancerogenic hypercycle‘ is also confirmed.

The fact of miRNA depression in a cancerous cell is also confirmed [21].

Therefore, there are at the present enough facts indicating a competing interaction between dsRNA RdRP and DNA world for the epigenetic control over the transcription and translation in a cell, and also indicating the fact that this control is, in a cancerous cell, under the regulation of a new RNA world order organizer represented by the dsRNA RdRP hypercycle. The quoted facts also indicate the displacing and replacing of miRNA by the product of the cancerous siRNA hypercycle, i. e., displacing and replacing of the DNA world by the RNA world.

The quoted facts are in favor of our hypothesis, but they cannot serve as its definite evidence. In general, our hypothesis cannot be proven based on a biochemical analysis method, i. e., method of separating of a whole system to its component elements. A cancerous hypercycle can be a quite complex emergence including several cyclic reactions linked to each other by hypercyclic links based on shared ferments as well as on RNA interference. A simple concentration evaluation of hypercycle components cannot provide us an image of the hypercycle as a dynamically developing structure.

As our hypothesis assumes the emergence of a new system from the elements of the precedent system, the proving of the hypothesis requires a synthesis method, a computer system modelling method, and comparison of this virtual model to the biological model.

For this, a biological model should be chosen an animal with a certain cancer form, the miRNA and siRNA concentrations in it as well as concentration of ferments replicating those RNAs should be examined, i. e., the biochemical profile of RNA and enzymes is to be examined. This profile should be compared to the correspondent profile of the control group of healthy animals. Based on the evaluated differences, a mathematical computer model of a cancerous hypercycle can be constructed and virtual experiments can be conducted, depressing the activity of ones or others enzymes of the hypercycle or modifying in a certain way other parameters of cyclic reactions (pH, concentration of chemical agents participating in the reaction and other). It should be mentioned that there is already experience of mathematical modelling of hypercycles [8]. Hence, it can be clarified which impact must be made on a cancerogenic hypercycle to create a Thom catastrophe with the goal to create a new dissipative system in which the DNA world would gain a selective advantage and prevail over the RNA world, and the emergence probability of this new dissipative system can also be calculated. Taking into account the gained result, the same action should be conducted on a real biological model and the gained results should be compared. The impact control and the evaluation of its effectiveness are conducted by scrutinizing the RNA profile and the enzymes. Taking into consideration the fact that the DNA methylation profile ("epigenetic code") in some mice tumours, e. g., such as bowel cancer, corresponds in a great measure to the DNA methylation image of the human bowel cancer, it is to be expected that the cancerogenic hypercycles structure determining such a similar "epigenetic code" in both cases will also be similar [22].

Applying such a method, several goals at one time can be achieved. The existence of a cancerous hypercycle can be proven as well as new possibilities for cancer diagnostics, prognosis and treatment can be detected.

4. Conclusion: New Conception of Cancer Treatment

Acting on the assumption of the hypothesis of cancer generation as a development of a cancerogenic hypercycle, we have to look differently at the impact mechanism of known anti-tumor treatment methods as well as on the cancer diagnostics and treatment strategy. The task of *diagnostics* becomes to detect the order parameters of the new dissipative system which the cancerous cell is. Such parameters are, most probably, siRNA, miRNA and activity of ferments strengthening the hypercycle.

The task of *treatment* becomes the creation of conditions in the cell that would change the competing interaction between the DNA world and the RNA world to a competing advantage in favor of the DNA world. This is the newness of the proposed cancer treatment conception and its difference from the modern cancer therapy: radical healing from cancer is impossible without elimination of the cancerous hypercycle.

Biochemical reactions run in a relatively narrow interval of physical and chemical parameters. To cause a selective effect with the goal of depressing one reaction and promoting the other one, it is necessary to know the difference of physical and chemical parameters of one reaction from those of the other one. Applied to our situation, it is necessary to know the difference of RNA replication parameters from the DNA replication parameters.

Target cancer therapy is aimed at elimination of consequences of expression of genes entailing uncontrollable cell division. Target therapy decelerates the development of a cancerogenic hypercycle by eliminating some of its components like e. g., expression of genes causing cell division, but it does not completely depress it as the primary cyclic RNA replication reaction continues to cause its impact on DNA methylation and on emergence of new DNA mutations.

This is why the main treatment targeted at restoration of the balance between the DNA and the RNA world has to be depression of the RNA world progression and, concretely, of one or another form of cancerogenic hypercycle.

The most logical and simplest method is blocking of activation of ferments replicating RNA RdRP. Amongst preparations able to cause such an impact is pyrogallol [23]. The anti-tumor impact of pyrogallol is already proven [24].

Elaboration of preparations causing selective depression of cancerogenic hypercycle enzymes can be a perspective direction in cancer treatment.

The cautious optimism in what concerns cancer treatment according to the proposed hypothesis of the cancerous hypercycle is caused by the fact that from ovules of mice to which nucleuses of cancer cells were transplanted, absolutely normal offspring was born. That is, replacing of the RNA world with destruction of the cancerous hypercycle in the cytoplasm entailed normalisation of the DNA world [25]. If we can destroy the cancerous hypercycle in the cell, we can also count on a positive result in cancer treatment.

References

[1] Hanahan D, Weinberg R.A *The Hallmarks of Cancer (review) Cell* 2000.v.100, p.57

[2] Setrov . I. General principles of systems organization and their methodological meaning. Leningrad, *"Science"* 1971, p.18

[3] Ashby R. U. An Introduction to cybernetics. Moscow, *"KomBook"*, 2005, p 432.

[4] Bogdanov A. A. Tectology: Universal organizational science. Moscow, *"Financiers"*, 2003, p. 273.

[5] Sedov . . *Informational-entropic features of social systems.* , nr. 5, 1993, p. 92-99 Available from: `http://ecsocman.hse.ru/data/149/386/1217/009_SEDOV.pdf`, last accessed 01.04.2014

[6] Zyrell S. “QWERTY effects”, “Path Dependence” and the law of hierarchical compensation. *Questions of economics*, nr. 8, 2005, p. 20 Available from: `http://ecsocman.hse.ru/text/16213158/`, last accessed 01.04.2014

[7] Are tumours a new species?. Bcking A Prof Dr mcd, Zylka-Mcnhorn V Dr med, *German Doctors journal* yr. 108, journal 48, (Deutsches rzteblatt Jg.108 Heft 48); 2011 Dec;A2604A2606

[8] Eigen M, Schuster P. The hypercycle. *A Principle of Natural Self-Organization.* Berlin Heidelberg New York, Moscow 1982: Springer Publishing House; 1979 [p. 1823, 7879, 175, 177].

[9] Spirin A.S. Protein bio-synthesis: regulation at the translation. *Soros Educ J* 2000;6(5):26.

[10] Starokadomsky P. Player Nr. 2 microRNA, *Biomolecule. A look from inside.* 2007-2012 biomolecule.ru, date of publication 9 June 2010, Available from: `http://biomolecula.ru/content/679`, last accessed 13.10.12.

[11] Sisken JE, Bonner SV, Grasch SD. *J Cell Physiol.* The prolongation of mitotic stages in SV40-transformed vs nontransformed human fibroblast cells. 1982 Nov;113(2):219-23.

[12] Khler Alwin, Hurt Ed. Gene regulation by nucleoporins and links to cancer. *Mol Cell* 2010;38(9):112.

[13] V. V. Isaeva. *Synergetics for biologists.* Vladivostok, 2003 pp. 7-26

[14] Rysnichenko G. Yu. Classis models of cell processes. on the website *‘Project mathematical cell* Project head Dr. phys. math. V. D. Lahno Available from:`http://www.mathcell.ru/ru/obzors/obzor_Rizn.shtml` last accessed 18.04.14

[15] Haken H. Success secrets of nature. *Synergetics: the teaching of coaction*, Moscow-Izhevsk, 2003, p. 9295, 99.

[16] Dymshits GM. Problem of restoration of DNA line molecules ends and telomerase. *Educ Magazine Soros* 2000;6(5):123.

[17] Bellare P, Sontheimer EJ. A fork in the road for microRNAs. *Nat Struct Mol Biol.* 2007 Aug;14(8): 6846

[18] Alexandrov AA Dr Biol Prof, editor. Knowledge base of molecular and general human biology (HUMBIO).Elaboration and realization. *RNA interference: RdRP activity in animals. secondary siRNAs.* Available from: `http://humbio.ru/humbio/rna_interf/00014f46.htm`; `http://humbio.ru/humbio/rna_interf/00012740.htm`, last accessed 15.08.2013

[19] Ting AH, Schuebel KE, Herman JG, Baylin JSB. Short double-stranded RNA induces transcriptional gene silencing in human cancer cells in the absence of DNA methylation. *Nat Genet.* 2005; Aug 37(8):90610.

[20] Morris KV, Chan SW, Jacobsen SE, Looney DJ. Small interfering RNA-induced transcriptional gene silencing in human cells. *Science.* 2004 Aug 27;305(5688):1289-92.

[21] Esquela-Kerscher A, Slack FJ. Oncomirs - microRNAs with a role in cancer. *Nat Rev Cancer.*2006 Apr;6(4):259-69

[22] Grimm C, Chavez L, Vilardell M, Farrall AL, Tierling S, Bhm JW, et al. DNAMethylome Analysis of Mouse Intestinal Adenoma Identifies a Tumour-Specific Signature That Is Partly Conserved in Human Colon Cancer. 2013.*PLoS Genet.* 9(2):e1003250. Available from: `http://www.plosgenetics.org/article/info`, last accessed 15.08.2013.

[23] M. V. Koslov MV, Polyakov KM, Ivanov AV, Filippova SE, Kusyakin AO, Tunitskaya VL, et al. RNA-dependent RNA polymerase of the hepatitis C virus: research of inhibiting mechanism of pyrogallolderivatives. *Biochemistry.*2006;71:Nr. 9, pp.12539.

[24] Yang CJ, Wang CS, Hung JY, Huang HW, Chia YC, Wang PH, et al. Pyrogallol induces G2-M arrest in human lung cancer cells and inhibits tumor growth in an animal model. *Lung Cancer*. 2009 Nov;66(2):1628.

[25] Illmensee K, Mintz B. Totipotency and normal differentiation of single teratocarcinoma cells cloned by injection into blastocysts. *Proc Natl Acad Sci* U S A. 1976 Feb;73(2):549-53.

In: Influenza and RNA Viruses
Editor: R. H. Bishop, pp. 55-77

ISBN: 978-1-63321-799-7

Chapter 3

MOLECULAR EPIDEMIOLOGY OF THE HUMAN-INFECTING INFLUENZA A VIRUS (H7N9) AND ITS POTENTIAL TO THE PANDEMICS

***Di Liu*[1,*], *Weifeng Shi*[2,3] and *Chen Chen*[4,5]**

[1]Network Information Center, Institute of Microbiology, Chinese Academy of Sciences, Beijing, China

[2]Collaborative Innovation Center for the Origin and Control of Emerging Infectious Diseases, Taishan Medical College, Shandong Province, China

[3]Institute of Pathogen Biology, Taishan Medical College, Shandong Province, China

[4]State Key Laboratory for Infectious Disease Prevention and Control National Institute for Communicable Disease Control and Prevention, Chinese Center for Disease Control and Prevention, Beijing, China

[5]Collaborative Innovation Center for Diagnosis and Treatment of Infectious Diseases, Hangzhou, China

* E-mail address: liud@im.ac.cn; Address: No.1 Beichen West Road, Chaoyang District, Beijing 100101, China (Corresponding Author).

Abstract

In the spring of 2013, the novel emerging influenza A (H7N9) virus has shocked China, and caused 134 human infections with 45 deaths in its first influenza season. In the winter of 2013-2014, the virus stroke China again and has caused 273 cases with 108 deaths (as of April 27th). The H7N9 outbreak has raised the concern of the next influenza pandemic. In this chapter, we briefly described the epidemiology of the H7N9 outbreak, and discussed the origin and diversity of the virus genome. Several models, including dynamic reassortments and genetic tuning models regarding the virus genesis, establishment and evolution were addressed. Moreover, we estimated and predicted the transmission routes of the H7N9 virus in China by means of big data. The co-circulation of H7N9 and varied subtypes of avian influenza viruses within poultry in China was described and discussed, as it is important for the establishment of the unpredictable HxNy influenza virus. Based on investigation of the molecular epidemiology of the H7N9 virus, the complete shutdown of the live poultry markets and firmly control of live poultry trade in China and Asian countries are called for to minimize avian influenza virus infections.

Introduction

Avian influenza virus is an important pathogen to both poultry industry and public health. Avian influenza virus belongs to the Influenza A Virus (species) of the Orthomyxoviridae family. The genome of influenza A virus consists of eight negative-sense single-stranded RNA segments, which encode 15 proteins to our current knowledge, of which four proteins (PA-X, PA-N155, PA-N182, and PB1-N40) were recently identified [1, 2]. Influenza A virus could be further classified into serotypes or subtypes according to its surface antigens, hemagglutinin (HA) and neuraminidase (NA), respectively. There are 16 serotypes of the HA and 9 serotypes of NA, and theoretically 144 HA-NA combinations in total (e.g., H1N1, H2N2, etc.). The HA protein functions as the recognition and binding to the receptors (sialylated lipids and/or proteins) of the susceptible cells [3]. The structural differences at the receptor-binding site of each subtype of HA determine the host-range of a given influenza virus, as mammalian hosts usually use the α2,6-linked sialic acids (α2,6SA) while the avian hosts favor α2,3-linked sialic acids (α2,3SA) to cell surface glycolipids or glycoproteins [4, 5]. However, amino acid substitutions at the receptor-binding site would greatly affect the binding affinity, and even cause the change from the binding to α2,3SA to α2,6SA, and vice versa [6-14].

Genetic reassortment is one of the most important features of the influenza virus. When two or more virus strains simultaneously infect one cell, they will replicate their genetic materials independently. However, budding viruses might randomly gain replicated gene segments and form novel virus strains (reassortants). After selections by hosts and transmission barriers, some of the novel reassortants might become prevalent. By means of genetic reassortment, influenza virus would easily gain novel genetic characterizations from other influenza viruses, in addition to the way of nucleotide substitutions. In particular, genetic reassortment between different subtypes of influenza A virus would generate novel subtype which has a mixture of surface antigens (HA and NA), and this is called antigenic shift. Reassortment of internal genes (PB2, PB1, PA, NP, M, and NS) would not cause antigenic shift, but would introduce amino acid substitutions that affect viral characters. For instance, the gain of Lysine at the position 627 of the PB2 protein will increase virus replication in mammalian hosts [15, 16].

It is generally believed that shorebirds and waterfowls act as natural reservoir for influenza virus, and nearly all subtypes of influenza virus have been discovered from them. Although the cross-species transmission of influenza viruses was limited by host receptors, virus adaptation and other aspects, many subtypes of influenza viruses have been found to infect poultry, pigs, cats, dogs and even human beings, including the highly pathogenic avian H5N1, the swine-origin pandemic H1N1 (pH1N1) and the avian-origin influenza A H7N9 virus that caused the 2013 and 2014 outbreaks in China. Recently, influenza-like viruses, H17N10 and H18N11, were identified from bats captured in Guatemala and Peru [17, 18]. The HA and NA proteins of bat-derived influenza viruses have displayed canonical structural modes, but lacking of the classical molecule functions [17, 19-23]. Though there is no report of the influenza A virus infection in bat, the discovery of influenza-like virus in bats raised the concerns of broader host ranges.

The H7N9 subtype of the influenza virus has been previously isolated from birds, and the genome sequences of H7N9 viruses could be traced back to 1988, from turkeys in Minnesota. After that, viruses from wild birds, including ruddy turnstone, mallard, blue-winged teal, and emperor goose, have been isolated and sequenced. The H7N9 subtype of influenza virus has been described from wild birds in America, Europe and Asia, but never found to infect mammals before 2013. Nevertheless, other H7 subtypes avian influenza viruses, including H7N1, H7N2, H7N3 and H7N7, have been reported to cause more than 100 human infections, among which a fatal case was reported in the Netherlands in 2003 [24-27]. The human infections of H7 avian influenza viruses have indicated that the H7 subtype has the ability to infect human; however, nobody had ever thought it would reassert with the N9 subtype and cause human infections in China.

In this chapter, we will look back to the H7N9 outbreaks in China of 2013 and 2014. The subjects will focus on the epidemiology, origin and diversity, dynamic reassortment and genetic tuning of the human-infecting H7N9 virus; and we will also address the environmental issues that 'inoculate' the H7N9 viruses, such as the live poultry markets and poultry transportation.

Epidemiology of the Human-Infecting H7N9 Virus

The first identified patient of H7N9 infection was an 87-year-old retired man, who had illness onset on February 18, 2013 in Shanghai municipal city, and admitted to hospital after one week. He had no known history of exposure to live birds two weeks before the onset. The second was a 27-year-old man, and the third was a 35-year-old housewife, both of whom had known contact to live birds [28]. These are the first three confirmed H7N9 infection cases, and the novel subtype of human-infecting influenza virus has reminded the world of threat of any combination of the influenza virus [29].

Until April 17, 2013, two months after the first H7N9 infection, a total of 82 confirmed cases emerged with a median age of 63-year-old [30]. The first five infections were all in Shanghai, implying the source of the H7N9 would be there. Most of these patients had known history of exposure to live chickens [30]. Within the first two months, the infections had been reported in six provinces and municipal cities. The virus kept spreading and causing human infections until summer came, as only occasional cases were reported from May to December 2013. Until December 1, 2013, the H7N9 virus has spread out to 12 provinces and municipal cities in Mainland China, including Shanghai, Anhui, Jiangsu, Zhejiang, Henan, Beijing, Shandong, Hebei, Jiangxi, Hunan, Fujian, and Guangdong, and caused 139 confirmed infections [30]. Taiwan and Hong Kong also reported infected patients who had traveled to Mainland China [31, 32]. 82% of these patients had a history of exposure to live animals. The surveillance of live poultry markets revealed potential poultry-to-human transmission [33, 34]. The closure of live poultry markets shortly after the H7N9 outbreak had markedly reduced the daily number of infections, based on an ecologic estimation [35].

More than one-third of the human infections are fatal. In 2013, 47 out of the 139, and in 2014, another 108 out of 273 infected humans died. In addition to those patients with severe lower respiratory tract illness, H7N9 infection could also cause mild symptoms. By means of the national influenza-like illness surveillance network, China CDC has revealed some cases with mild illness [36]. This finding revealed broader clinical spectrum of the H7N9 infection, and had implied the underestimation of the H7N9 infection numbers in China. A further assessment estimated about 27,000 people had been infected by the H7N9 virus [33]. Until now, no conclusively established human-to-human transmission was observed, although in several families reported limited, non-sustained human-to-human transmissions [30].

Origin of the Human-Infecting H7N9 Virus

Tracing the origin of a pathogen is of vital importance for its prevention and control. Shortly after the first human-infecting H7N9 influenza virus was confirmed on March 30, 2013, a number of studies were conducted to identify the potential origin of this novel strain. Based on the comparison of the full-genome sequence of this virus and associated virus sequences searched from GenBank through BLAST [37], the origin of this virus was undoubtedly pointed to avian hosts from the very beginning of the outbreak, and its correlation between H7N9 viruses isolated from live poultry markets indicated the poultry-to-human transmission route. [28, 33, 34, 38].

The first report on the origin of the novel human-infecting H7N9 influenza virus proposed that each of the eight gene segments was of avian origin [28]. From the phylogenetic trees, the HA gene was close to those from duck H7N3 influenza viruses isolated from Zhejiang Province of China, while the NA gene was closely adjacent to the H7N9 influenza viruses isolated from wild birds from South Korea. The internal genes were highly similar to those of avian H9N2 influenza viruses circulating in China. Interestingly, three of the internal genes, PB2, PB1, and PA, were very close to those of an H9N2 strain isolated from a brambling in Beijing (A/brambling/ Beijing/16/2012(H9N2), abbreviated as BJ16). Initially, the H7N3 from ducks, H7N9 from wild migratory birds, and H9N2 from bramblings, were considered as the genetic sources of the human-infecting H7N9 virus [28].

Then questions were raised as how did the influenza viruses from these birds meet and reassort between each other, and which would be the intermediate host? To answer theses question, more comprehensive phylogenetic and coalescence analyses were performed. And the migratory flyway of wild birds, the habitats of wild and domestic waterfowls, and the probable connections between each host were considered to interpret the phylogenetic trees of each gene. In detail, the HA gene fell within the Eurasian lineage of H7 and the most closely related strain was isolated from ducks from Zhejiang Province in 2011. This observation is in accordance with previous reports [28, 38]. Further inspection of the H7 phylogeny revealed that different H7 viruses have been circulating among wild ducks in Eastern China, South Korea and Japan, which were located along the East Asian flyway. In addition, viral transmission from wild birds to domestic ducks has also been observed. These observations indicate that H7 subtype influenza viruses from wild birds are occasionally transmitted to domestic waterfowls along the migratory flyways. The estimated time to most recent common ancestor (tMRCA) of the novel H7N9 strains was around January 2012 (Mean, January, 2012; 95% HPD: March, 2011–October, 2012). At that time, wild birds were wintering in southern China. Therefore, it was possible that wild birds spread the H7 influenza viruses to domestic ducks and these corresponding H7 strains had been circulating in ducks for at least one year before causing human infections [39].

Likewise, the NA gene of an H7N9 virus isolated from wild ducks from South Korea was found to be the most related sequence for the novel H7N9 viruses. These viruses were collected in February and April of 2011, respectively, and the estimated tMRCA of the NA gene was in approximately mid-June of 2011 (Mean: June, 2011; 95% HPD: March, 2010 –July, 2012). However, at that time, these birds might have just arrived in South Korea for breeding from Southeast China along the East Asian flyway. Therefore, these birds might have transmitted the viruses to birds or domestic ducks when they flied northwards along eastern China, as they have similar behaviors and share habitats with local waterfowls in Eastern China. And then reassortment between avian influenza viruses carried by ducks or chickens gave rise to the H7HA and N9NA to the novel H7N9 influenza virus, although whether such reassortment events occurring in ducks or chickens remain unknown. In addition, the possibility of the existence of certain intermediate hosts was also indicated by the long-branch between the novel H7N9 and other influenza virus isolates from wild birds in the tree [39].

However, regarding the origin of the internal genes, slight difference existed. On one hand, all the internal gene segments of the human-infecting influenza viruses were closely related to those from avian H9N2 viruses, particularly BJ16 collected on November 7th, 2012 [28]. Brambling is a migratory bird and may fly southwards for wintering. It is possible that brambling brings this virus from northern China (Beijing) to southern China (Shanghai) and leads to the genesis of the novel H7N9 influenza virus. However, on the other hand, by close inspection of the phylogenetic trees, we found that in the NP, M and NS trees, the novel H7N9 influenza viruses did not cluster together with BJ16. Alternatively, they are more closely related to chicken-origin H9N2 viruses. Furthermore, although in the trees of PB2, PB1 and PA, the novel H7N9 influenza viruses did form an independent sub-lineage with BJ16, there is a relatively long branch length gap between them. In addition, whether brambling can possess a virus population big enough to act as the source of the H7N9 influenza virus remains unknown, because only one strain was isolated from brambling based on current surveillance data. The estimated time to most recent common ancestor (tMRCA) of three polymerase genes were dated before June of 2012, suggesting the brambling H9N2 virus is a newer strain than to be the ancestor of the novel human-infecting H7N9 virus. Hence, we favored an alternative explanation that the three-polymerase genes, as well as the other internal genes might probably come from H9N2 viruses from chicken populations, though the possibility that wild birds have brought earlier lineages of viruses to Southern China cannot be fully excluded.

Almost at the same time, Chen and colleagues successfully isolated several H7N9 influenza viruses from chickens from live poultry market and found that they were highly similar to those isolated from humans in the eight gene segments [33]. Based on this finding, they also proposed an avian-origin of the human-infecting influenza viruses, which was consistent with our result obtained from coalescent analysis.

To conclude, the HA gene might come from AIVs of duck origin, and the NA gene might be originally derived from AIVs from migratory birds along the East Asian flyway. The six internal genes of this virus most likely originated from H9N2 influenza viruses isolated from chickens. Although it remains unknown that the final reassortment event giving rise to the novel H7N9 influenza virus occurs in ducks or chickens, they probably acted as the intermediate hosts leading to the origin of the lethal H7N9 virus.

Phylogenetic Diversity of the H7N9 Virus

The diversity of the H7N9 influenza virus has been noticed by inspections of the first four virus strains; A/Anhui/1/2013 (AH/1), A/Shanghai/2/2013 (SH/2) and A/Hangzhou/1/2013 (HZ/1) clustered into a lineage, while A/Shanghai/1/2013 (SH/1) fell outside judging from the H7 phylogeny [28, 33, 39]. Similar phylogeny was also observed in the NA phylogenetic tree. In addition, the internal gene, NP, also presented a certain divergence, whereas SH/1 was clustered together with A/chicken/Shanghai/C1/2012(H9N2) [39, 40]. Subsequently, as more human infection cases with H7N9 influenza viruses were confirmed and more virus sequences were available in public database, Zhang et al. reported that the PB2, PB1, PA, and M genes have also formed at least two clusters in the phylogenetic trees [40]. Based on a phylogenetic analysis of 45 H7N9 and 42 H9N2 viruses isolated from various hosts recently, Wu et al. also classified the H7N9 influenza viruses into two clusters for PB2, PB1, PA, NP and M genes, one consisting of more sequences and named as major cluster and the other named as minor cluster [41]. Based on this designation, they classified the 45 H7N9 viruses into nine genotypes.

Our team and collaborators collected a total of 109 H7N9 viruses with 89 full-length genome sequences and found that all the six internal genes have presented certain genetic diversity [42]. Furthermore, according to the bootstrap value (>75) and the branch length (>0.001), we classified each viral gene into various clades and established a nomenclature system for the H7N9 viruses. In this nomenclature system, if all internal genes fell into the major clade (clade 1 or 1.1), the genotype of this virus was assigned as G0. If strains have one internal gene different from G0 in the phylogenetic classification, they were assigned as genotype G1, and so on. Therefore, strains with all six internal genes different from G0 were assigned as G6. Within each of the G1–G6 series, genotypes were further assigned (for example, G2.1) if any two internal genes came from a different origin. Based on this rule, a total of 27 different genotypes were identified. In particular, different to previous influenza viruses, such as pandemic H1N1 (2009) and highly pathogenic H5N1 avian influenza viruses, which HA genes were more diversified than the internal genes, the internal genes of the H7N9 influenza viruses showed a more diversified feature. All these suggest that the H7N9 viruses of this outbreak might be largely diversified to what we observed from previous studies.

Models of the H7N9 Formation and Reassortments

With regard to how the H7N9 viruses construct their genetic constellation, a number of models have been proposed. The first model believed that the novel H7N9 influenza virus was produced via three reassortment events. The HA gene might be originated from duck H7 influenza virus, while the NA gene might be originated from a strain isolated from a wild bird in South Korea. The internal genes of the H7N9 viruses might be derived from a strain from brambling, BJ16 [28].

Improved from the initial model, the second model proposed that four reassortment events gave rise to the human-infecting H7N9 influenza virus. Similarly, the HA gene might come from duck H7 influenza virus and the NA gene might be originally derived from a wild bird strain. However, the NA gene might be transferred to a poultry host (most possibly, duck) first before causing human infection, in spite of lack of direct surveillance data. In addition, the internal genes might have two independent sources, with the NS gene coming from a source and the remaining genes from another source [39].

Subsequently, Wu and colleagues proposed a sequential reassortment model, in which the H7N9 viruses were generated by at least two-step sequential reassortments [41]. The first reassortment event likely occurred in wild birds, and the viruses obtained the HA and NA genes. The second might occur in domestic birds, and the viruses obtained their internal genes. In the second step, genetically distinct H9N2 viruses acted as genetic donors for the H7N9 viruses.

Thereafter, Cui et al. performed a comprehensive analysis of the H7N9 viruses in the spring outbreak in 2013 and proposed a dynamic reassortment model [42]. In this model, after the H7N9 viruses obtained the HA and NA genes, they obtained the internal genes through dynamic reassortment with local H9N2 influenza viruses. This process occurs with the virus spread via inter-province poultry transportation. This model explains why there are so many H7N9 genotypes and how they were generated.

More recently, Wang and colleagues analyzed the amino acid polymorphism of a total of 146 full-length human and non-human H7N9 influenza virus genomes and proposed a genetic tuning model from the perspective of molecular characterization [43]. In this report, the authors described a prototype H7N9 strain, A/Shanghai/05/2013(H7N9) (SH/5). Different from other H7N9 influenza viruses identified in this outbreak, the HA and NA gene of this strain always fell outside the major H7N9 lineage in the tree, formed an outgroup. In particular, this strain had totally avian-like genetic signatures, such as HA 186G and 226Q, and long NA stalk. Then this strain gave rise to SH/1-like strains, which possess HA 186G and 226Q, and a truncated NA stalk. Then A/Shanghai/1/2013(H7N9)-like strains produced AH/1-like strains, with HA 186V and 226L, and a truncated NA stalk. The HA 186V and 226L are human-like genetic signatures. It should be also noted that AH/1 is the prototype strain for genotype G0, which was the prevalent genotype in the 2013 spring outbreak and was responsible for the spread of the H7N9 virus in China [42]. Then the AH/1-like strains recruited various internal genes and formed the diversified H7N9 genotypes. The final step of this genetic tuning process was the gain of PB2 627K and 701N, which enhanced viral replication efficiency in the upper respiratory tract of mammalian hosts.

Molecular Characterizations of the H7N9 Virus

Molecular characterization analysis of the viral genomes could provide insight into viral features, such as pathogenicity, host receptor preference, and drug resistance.

The number of basic amino acids at the cleavage site between HA1 and HA2 has been found to be vital for viral pathogenicity [44]. In the first three H7N9 virus strains, only one basic amino acid, R (Arginine), was identified at the cleavage site of the HA protein. Further analysis of the H7N9 viruses isolated subsequently failed to find multiple basic amino acids at the connecting site. This suggested that the novel H7N9 influenza virus was low pathogenic to poultry.

It has been proved that the glutamine (Q) to Leucine (L) substitution at position 226 (H3 numbering) at the receptor-binding site might cause virus high-affinity binding to human receptor [45]. At this position, the H7N9 influenza viruses presented certain amino acid polymorphism. Only a few viruses possess Q, while most of them possess L at this position, whatever they were isolated from human or poultry. This suggested the majority of the H7N9 viruses might prefer to attach human receptors. In addition, the substitution Q217I (Isoleucine) was also observed, for example, A/Hangzhou/1/2013, which probably had the potential for high-affinity binding to human receptor due to the similar hydrophobic nature to Leucine [39].

A deletion in the NA stalk has been described to facilitate type A influenza to better adapt to terrestrial poultry after introduction from aquatic birds [46-48]. This deletion has been previously found in influenza A H5N1 [46], H9N2[49], H7 [50], as well as the novel H7N9 virus [28]. Further study showed that all the isolates present in this study possessed a five-amino acid-deletion (from position 69 to 73) in the NA stalk, indicating that the novel H7N9 virus has gained better adaptation to terrestrial environment.

Multiple substitutions in the polymerase-coding genes have also been reported to be associated with enhanced polymerase activity of type A influenza, such as PB2 E627K, PB2 D701N, PB2 714R, PA 615R, and NP 319K [16, 51, 52]. Among the H7N9 strains, approximately one third of them held PB2 627K and a small number of them held PB2 701N, while none of them possessed PB2 714R, PA 615R and NP 319K. Interestingly, the PB2 E627K has seldom been seen in avian influenza A (H9N2) viruses, where the PB2 gene is derived in the dynamic reassorting process, suggesting that it might be a novel adaptive mutation obtained shortly after introduction into humans.

In particular, a number of amino acids have been associated with conferring drug resistance to the influenza virus. For example, the 294K (292 in N2 numbering) in the NA protein has been found to confer resistance to oseltamivir [53, 54]. Sequence analyses have shown that none of the virus strains held 294K in the NA protein, except for SH/1. This is in agreement with the finding that viruses holding the substitution 294K in the NA protein might have less fitness [55]. Clinically, in a few patients, the R292K substitution may be produced after 2 days antiviral treatment[56].The Ser31Asn substitution in the M2 protein confers virus resistance to adamantanes [57]. Unfortunately, all the novel H7N9 influenza viruses possessed 32Asn, which suggested they have had resistance to adamantanes [33].

Depicting Poultry Transportation Network through the Online Knowledge

The H7N9 virus was clearly of avian origin and the live poultry markets were considered as the major areas to exchange the viral isolates [58]. Most of patients had a history of exposure to live animals [30]. No obvious evidence has proven the virus can be transmitted from human to human efficiently. Thus, live poultry are the major infection sources of the H7N9 virus, and its travelling and transferring among provinces would cause virus spreading [59]. Therefore, it would be possible to estimate the spreading of H7N9 by detecting and tracking the movement of live birds in live poultry markets.

Large scale online knowledge has been proven to be a powerful tool to investigate the social phenomena associated with infectious diseases. US CDC and GOOGLE developed a website to predict the flu outbreak, which may find an outbreak a week earlier than traditional disease report system [60, 61] (http://www.google.org/flutrends/). The daily incidence of H5N1 virus outbreaks in Vietnam peaks around the annual holiday festivities in February is also detected by big data from Internet [62, 63].

Serials of open source script which can collect the public online information, and keywords (city name) and (live poultry) and (exchange or carrier) with the similar meaning local language were used. These keywords are with the following format: (city name) and (live poultry or poultry or pigeon or quail or birds or migratory bird or chicken or duck or goose) and (come from or exchange or source or carrier or travel or supply or market or slaughter house or production area). The pages that fit our format were included in the hash list. In our analysis, we integrated the following algorithm and model, including PageRank algorithm, BloomFilter, SVM model and ZooKeeper, to automatically control the downloading, analyze the information and manage the numeric process [64, 65].

The webpages associated to H7N9 infections were considered, in order to examine the source of H7N9. Before May 7, 2013, a total of 835,635 webpages were crawled from Internet and 2943 pages were of interest, in which 922 pages contained live poultry trading information of Shanghai [66, 67]. Following the processes of qualification and removing redundancy, a total of 315 queries with the exact trading information among the cities by crowd-powered method were created at the urgent period. The trade links among cities were distilled from the above two sources, when these cities occurred in one webpage or query, containing 25,942 information based connections (IC) and 591 context based connections (CC). Based on the connections, the force direct graphs were constructed at the province level and the city level to study the nationwide live poultry-trading route.

The graphs clearly implicated that the live birds in Shanghai were traded from Jiangsu, Zhejiang and Anhui provinces. In the 682 live bird-trading queries of Shanghai, 84% (571) were linked with Jiangsu, Zhejiang and Anhui provinces. Shanghai authority stated that approximately 80% live birds in this city were from the above three provinces. Therefore, live birds from those three provinces and Shanghai were considered as potential infectious sources for the new infection. The H7N9 epidemiology has noted the date of onset illness of the first patient in Shanghai was February 18, and those of the first patient in Zhejiang, Jiangsu and Anhui province were March 7, 15 and 19, respectively. On April 7, Shanghai, Jiangsu, Zhejiang and Anhui established the Joint Prevention and Control Mechanism and started to close live poultry markets. Therefore, two stages could be designated during the H7N9 outbreak. Before the closure of live poultry markets, the public was unaware of the poultry-to-human transmission; and after that live birds trading activities had been markedly affected, and people were asked to keep away from live poultry markets. During the first stage, 106 people from 11 prefecture-level cities were infected. In the second stage, the infected prefecture-level cities increased to 28, covering 11 county-level cities, implying the H7N9 virus had spread out by means of poultry transportation. However, the number of infected humans was 22. It was clear that the first wave was characterized as more people infected, and the second wave was featured as more cities infected, indicating live bird trading contributed to the geographic extension of the viral pathogen.

We draw the topological map of H7N9 virus spreading at the province and city levels based on live bird trading information. The province risk of H7N9 was estimated by the live birds trading connections to the first wave provinces, including Shanghai, Zhejiang, Jiangsu and Anhui. We have not found any connections of the first wave provinces with 8 provinces, indicating that they have no or very low risk of H7N9 infections by live bird trading, namely Jilin, Gansu, Qinghai, Inner Mongolia, Henan, Yunnan, Heilongjiang provinces, Tianjin and Chongqing cities. Among them, Qinghai only had live bird trade information on context, while we do not find any connection in crawled pages. Of 18 provinces suggested as the high-risk group, 10 were infected, having patients diagnosed. It should mention that a patient diagnosed in Taiwan had travelled to Jiangsu province previously. No connection was observed for 5 provinces including Xinjiang, Ningxia, Tibet, Guizhou, Shaanxi, as well as Hong Kong, Macao and Taiwan. Therefore, there should be no risk for them to have infection of H7N9 by live bird trading, based on our analysis. However, few data can be found to illustrate the transfer route among all cities. An exception appears in the Southeast China, where locates the relative rich cities. However, this outbreak region is overlapped with this region. Thus, we may estimate the possible transfer route among the major cities. The transfer map of the cities has been drawn in our analysis [67].

The topological map has no direction, and it is hard to evaluate the transmission directions. Thus, together with the time order of the cities infected, we proposed three major routes of the H7N9 spread. The first one is associated with the infection strain in Beijing. The most probable route is by live birds carrying virus from Chuzhou of Anhui or Yancheng of Jiangsu province. Epidemiological data supports this hypothesis that the two cities were infected in 9 March or 8 April respectively, earlier than Beijing (April 11). The second showed that Chuzhou of Anhui might be infected by live birds carrying viruses from Hangzhou of Zhejiang province or Shanghai. It was also supported by the epidemiological data that Chuzhou was infected later than Hangzhou and Shanghai. Surprised enough, the genome sequences of the virus strain isolated from patient from Chuzhou were highly homologous with those of strains isolated from patients and chickens from Hangzhou, and from one of two isolates from patients in Shanghai (1, 2). The last route showed that Nanchang city of Jiangxi province and Fuzhou city of Fujian province were probable infected by viruses from live birds traded from Shanghai. Both cities were accordingly infected later than Shanghai.

After the first H7N9 outbreak in Apr to May of 2013, another outbreak peak appears in January 2, 2014 to February 27, 2014. During this period, the H7N9 virus infected 202 people. Different from the first outbreak, the hotspot of the infection region is southern china, and Guangdong is the major province. Although the topologic transfer map of the live poultry is almost the same, the potential infection risk of province was different because their orient of the outbreak sites was different.

Compare to traditional investigation of H7N9, our analysis by using big data from website is cheap, fast and easy to carry out, and it will not be affected by the bias of sampling, and the information hidden during the outbreak period. However, its limitations are also obvious. First, the limited knowledge or data would mislead us to identify the inappropriate target of virus infection. For example, it is hard to find the exact transfer route for several cities, where have limited information on the web, such as cities in Tibet or Guizhou province. Second, the noise of the data is large, and we have no useful methods to identify this information. Generally, we will use keywords to seek the spread of the disease only when the outbreak occurred. However, obtaining all information from websites without selection needs a large amount of resources of network, time cost as well as hard disk area. Fortunately, little information about H7N9 or similar words appears in Internet due to specific proper name at the beginning of the outbreak.

Co-circulated Avian Influenza Viruses in CHINA

During the past ten years, numerous avian influenza subtypes have been identified in China, though the avian influenza surveillance system has not been fully established. For instance, H5N1 [68], H9N2 [69], and H6N1 [70, 71] have been found to circulating in poultry in China in a long term. In particular, since February 2013, four subtypes have been identified to cause human infection, H7N9 [28], H6N1 [72], H10N8 [73], and H5N6 (http://www.chinadaily.com.cn/china/2014-05/09/content_17496951.htm). So far, it has come to the consensus that there is a huge influenza pool in China.

In Chinese poultry populations (particularly chickens), H9N2 influenza viruses have been circulating more than twenty years [69, 74], and they have been isolated from almost all provinces in recent years. It is low pathogenic to poultry, and poultry with this viral infection often show no or slight symptoms. Therefore, the transmission of this virus is likely to have been neglected through poultry transportations. Extensive and prolonged circulation has made H9N2 influenza viruses very diversified and viruses from different regions often have certain region-specific genetic characterizations. This also leads to the co-circulation of numerous genotypes in China. It is the diversified H9N2 influenza viruses that act as genetic donors for the novel H7N9 influenza viruses and are responsible for the diversified internal genes of H7N9 viruses obtained through dynamic reassortment [42]. A recent study also reveals that the novel human-infecting H10N8 influenza virus also adopts internal genes from H9N2 viruses and might be also undergoing a similar dynamic reassortment process like H7N9 [75]. This highlights that further attention should be made to monitor the evolution and variation of the novel H7N9 and H10N8 influenza viruses.

Another influenza virus circulating in China for almost twenty years is highly pathogenic H5N1 influenza virus [68]. Because of its high pathogenicity to chickens, ducks act as the major hosts for H5N1. This is different from H9N2, which mainly circulate in chickens. Current surveillance has revealed that there are several combinations with H5 and different NA subtypes in China, such as H5N1, H5N2, H5N6, and H5N8. In addition, reassortments between H5 influenza viruses with other subtypes have been frequently described both in poultry and swine, especially with H9N2 [49].

The third major subtype circulated in China is H6. Viruses of H6 subtype have been isolated from various hosts in live poultry markets [76], such as chickens, ducks [77], and minor poultry species [70, 78]. They were also low pathogenic to poultry; however, they were regarded as candidates to potentially cause influenza pandemics approximately one third of the tested viruses could recognize human-type receptor, and almost all the viruses tested could replicate efficiently in the lungs in mice [71]. In addition, a half of tested viruses could be transmitted to contacted guinea pigs. H6 also undergoes frequent reassortments with other subtypes. An H6N1 influenza virus has been once regarded as the internal gene donors of H5N1 [79]. In addition, a few internal genes of the human-infecting H6N1 influenza virus identified in Taiwan were highly similar to those of the H5N2 subtype [72, 80].

In November 2013, a novel H10N8 influenza virus caused human infection in Jiangxi Province [73]. Phylogenetic analysis has shown that its internal genes were also derived from the H9N2 influenza viruses. Subsequently, more H10N8 influenza viruses were isolated from chickens and environmental samples in Jiangxi (Unpublished data). Their HA and NA genes were similar to those of the human isolate, whereas they had different internals genes. Therefore, we speculate that the novel H10N8 might have become established among chickens and might also undergo a similar dynamic reassortment process like H7N9.

Apart from the subtypes mentioned above, some other subtypes have also been detected in China [74]. The existence and co-circulation of these identified subtypes and potentially unidentified subtypes make China become a huge influenza pool, which makes it extremely difficult to predict which combination of HA and NA would cause the next influenza pandemic.

Although the causes shaping the genetic diversity of the influenza pool have not been well understood, a number of factors might contribute to the genetic complexity of this influenza pool. First, there are several migration pathways of wild birds in China. Every year, millions of wild birds fly southward for wintering and fly back for breeding, by way of China. Many lakes in eastern China provide birds freshwater and act as stopovers for birds. This enhances the possibility of virus transfer from wild birds to domestic birds. Second, poultry industry of China is very prosperous. Approximately half of worldwide ducks are raised in China [81]. Duck can shed high-titer viruses for a few days and act as viral source. Third, poultry transportation network of China is very complex and this facilitates virus spread [67]. Last but not least, the segmented genome of type A influenza facilitates genetic exchange between different influenza subtypes via a genetic mechanism, reassortment. Genetic reassortment may produce influenza variants with novel genetic, antigenic and viral features.

Conclusion

In summary, the human-infecting influenza A (H7N9) virus was an avian-origin influenza virus, and possibly experienced sequential genetic reassortments among wild birds, domestic ducks and poultry. During the interspecies transmission, the H7N9 virus has evolved its genome step by step to adapt to the hosts, from the wild birds to domestic birds, and from waterfowls to terrestrial poultry. As the H7N9 virus was low pathogenic to poultry, the spread of H7N9 via poultry transportation has made it hidden within the poultry of most areas in China, like the prevalent H9N2 virus. By means of dynamic reassortments with poultry H9N2 influenza viruses the H7N9 virus has gained the ability to genetically tune its genome to adapt to varied hosts. The receptor-binding affinity of the HA showed that the H7N9 virus could attach to the mammalian receptors, but distinct from that of a human virus. So that sustained human-to-human transmissions have not been identified yet.

The emergence of the novel H7N9 virus re-opened the awareness that what HxNy would be the next, and could it be an influenza pandemic [29]? The establishment of the H7N9 virus also noted the public that the low pathogenic avian influenza virus circulating in poultry would also become fatal to humans. Not only the pigs, which have been considered as the mixing vessels, but also the birds themselves, especially poultry could act as the mixing vessels to incubate human/mammalian-infecting avian influenza viruses [82, 83]. As a tradition, Chinese and other Asian peoples are willing to enjoy the fresh meat right after the slaughtering of living animals; therefore live animal markets are very popular. The prosperity of those live animal markets grants avian influenza viruses great opportunity to evolve to adapt to new hosts and to transmit across interspecies barriers. For this purpose, closure of live animal markets, at least firmly control of live poultry trade, has urgently been proposed to prevent potential infection of avian influenza virus [84]. Besides live poultry trade, live poultry transportation played an important role in the spreading of avian influenza viruses. Transportations to and from small poultry farms are hardly to track using traditional methods. However, Internet has provided another way, as poultry owners and/or traders would post related information to their blogs or micro-blog (twitter-like system in Chinese) unintendedly. Attempts have showed that applying the information crawled from the Internet would be helpful to track and predict the spreading of avian influenza virus [67]. In addition to virus surveillance and phylogenetic, big data from Internet would be another pole to support the research of avian influenza viruses.

Acknowledgments

DL was supported by grants of China Ministry of Science and Technology Project 973 (grant no. 2010CB530303) and the intramural special grant for influenza virus research from the Chinese Academy of Sciences (KSZD-EW-Z-002). WS was supported by the Doctoral Starting Up Foundation of Taishan Medical College and a grant from the International Development Research Centre (IDRC). CC was supported by grants of China Ministry of Science and Technology Project 863 (2014AA021505) and Mega Project of Research on the Prevention and Control of HIV/AIDS, Viral Hepatitis Infectious Diseases (2013ZX10004-101).

Reference

[1] Wise, H.M., et al., A complicated message: Identification of a novel PB1-related protein translated from influenza A virus segment 2 mRNA. *J Virol,* 2009. 83(16): p. 8021-31.

[2] Muramoto, Y., et al., Identification of novel influenza A virus proteins translated from PA mRNA. *J Virol*, 2013. 87(5): p. 2455-62.

[3] Webster, R.G., et al., Evolution and ecology of influenza A viruses. *Microbiol Rev,* 1992. 56(1): p. 152-79.

[4] Wilson, I.A., J.J. Skehel, and D.C. Wiley, Structure of the haemagglutinin membrane glycoprotein of influenza virus at 3 A resolution. *Nature,* 1981. 289(5796): p. 366-73.

[5] Skehel, J.J. and D.C. Wiley, Receptor binding and membrane fusion in virus entry: the influenza hemagglutinin. *Annu Rev Biochem,* 2000. 69: p. 531-69.
[6] Wiley, D.C. and J.J. Skehel, The structure and function of the hemagglutinin membrane glycoprotein of influenza virus. *Annu Rev Biochem,* 1987. 56: p. 365-94.
[7] Liu, J., et al., Structures of receptor complexes formed by hemagglutinins from the Asian Influenza pandemic of 1957. *Proc Natl Acad Sci* U S A, 2009. 106(40): p. 17175-80.
[8] Zhang, W., et al., Molecular basis of the receptor binding specificity switch of the hemagglutinins from both the 1918 and 2009 pandemic influenza A viruses by a D225G substitution. *J Virol,* 2013. 87(10): p. 5949-58.
[9] Gamblin, S.J., et al., The structure and receptor binding properties of the 1918 influenza hemagglutinin. *Science,* 2004. 303(5665): p. 1838-42.
[10] Zhang, W., et al., An airborne transmissible avian influenza H5 hemagglutinin seen at the atomic level. *Science,* 2013. 340(6139): p. 1463-7.
[11] Xiong, X., et al., Receptor binding by an H7N9 influenza virus from humans. *Nature,* 2013. 499(7459): p. 496-9.
[12] Xiong, X., et al., Receptor binding by a ferret-transmissible H5 avian influenza virus. *Nature,* 2013. 497(7449): p. 392-6.
[13] Shi, Y., et al., Structures and receptor binding of hemagglutinins from human-infecting H7N9 influenza viruses. *Science,* 2013. 342(6155): p. 243-7.
[14] Lu, X., et al., Structure and receptor-binding properties of an airborne transmissible avian influenza A virus hemagglutinin H5 (VN1203mut). *Protein Cell,* 2013. 4(7): p. 502-11.
[15] Jonges, M., et al., Emergence of the virulence-associated PB2 E627K substitution in a fatal human case of highly pathogenic avian influenza virus A(H7N7) infection as determined by Illumina ultra-deep sequencing. *J Virol,* 2014. 88(3): p. 1694-702.
[16] Shinya, K., et al., PB2 amino acid at position 627 affects replicative efficiency, but not cell tropism, of Hong Kong H5N1 influenza A viruses in mice. *Virology,* 2004. 320(2): p. 258-66.
[17] Tong, S., et al., New world bats harbor diverse influenza A viruses. *PLoS Pathog,* 2013. 9(10): p. e1003657.
[18] Tong, S., et al., A distinct lineage of influenza A virus from bats. *Proc Natl Acad Sci* U S A, 2012. 109(11): p. 4269-74.

[19] Zhu, X., et al., Hemagglutinin homologue from H17N10 bat influenza virus exhibits divergent receptor-binding and pH-dependent fusion activities. *Proc Natl Acad Sci* U S A, 2013. 110(4): p. 1458-63.

[20] Sun, X., et al., Bat-derived influenza hemagglutinin H17 does not bind canonical avian or human receptors and most likely uses a unique entry mechanism. *Cell Rep,* 2013. 3(3): p. 769-78.

[21] Zhu, X., et al., Crystal structures of two subtype N10 neuraminidase-like proteins from bat influenza A viruses reveal a diverged putative active site. *Proc Natl Acad Sci* U S A, 2012. 109(46): p. 18903-8.

[22] Garcia-Sastre, A., The neuraminidase of bat influenza viruses is not a neuraminidase. *Proc Natl Acad Sci* U S A, 2012. 109(46): p. 18635-6.

[23] Wu, Y., et al., Bat-derived influenza-like viruses H17N10 and H18N11. *Trends Microbiol,* 2014. 22(4): p. 183-91.

[24] Nguyen-Van-Tam, J.S., et al., Outbreak of low pathogenicity H7N3 avian influenza in UK, including associated case of human conjunctivitis. *Euro Surveill,* 2006. 11(5): p. E060504 2.

[25] Fouchier, R.A., et al., Avian influenza A virus (H7N7) associated with human conjunctivitis and a fatal case of acute respiratory distress syndrome. *Proc Natl Acad Sci* U S A, 2004. 101(5): p. 1356-61.

[26] Stegeman, A., et al., Avian influenza A virus (H7N7) epidemic in The Netherlands in 2003: course of the epidemic and effectiveness of control measures. *J Infect Dis,* 2004. 190(12): p. 2088-95.

[27] Avian influenza A/(H7N2) outbreak in the United Kingdom. *Euro Surveill,* 2007. 12(5): p. E070531 2.

[28] Gao, R., et al., Human infection with a novel avian-origin influenza A (H7N9) virus. *N Engl J Med,* 2013. 368(20): p. 1888-97.

[29] Wu, Y. and G.F. Gao, Lessons learnt from the human infections of avian-origin influenza A H7N9 virus: live free markets and human health. *Sci China Life Sci,* 2013. 56(6): p. 493-4.

[30] Li, Q., et al., Epidemiology of human infections with avian influenza A(H7N9) virus in China. *N Engl J Med,* 2014. 370(6): p. 520-32.

[31] Chang, S.Y., et al., The first case of H7N9 influenza in Taiwan. *Lancet,* 2013. 381(9878): p. 1621.

[32] To, K.K., et al., Unique reassortant of influenza A(H7N9) virus associated with severe disease emerging in Hong Kong. *J Infect,* 2014. 69(1): p. 60-8.

[33] Chen, Y., et al., Human infections with the emerging avian influenza A H7N9 virus from wet market poultry: clinical analysis and characterisation of viral genome. *Lancet,* 2013. 381(9881): p. 1916-25.

[34] Shi, J.Z., et al., Isolation and characterization of H7N9 viruses from live poultry markets-Implication of the source of current H7N9 infection in humans. *Chinese Science Bulletin,* 2013. 58(16): p. 1857-1863.

[35] Yu, H., et al., Effect of closure of live poultry markets on poultry-to-person transmission of avian influenza A H7N9 virus: an ecological study. *Lancet,* 2014. 383(9916): p. 541-8.

[36] Xu, C., et al., Monitoring avian influenza A(H7N9) virus through national influenza-like illness surveillance, China. *Emerg Infect Dis,* 2013. 19(8): p. 1289-92.

[37] Altschul, S.F., et al., Basic local alignment search tool. *J Mol Biol,* 1990. 215(3): p. 403-10.

[38] Kageyama, T., et al., Genetic analysis of novel avian A(H7N9) influenza viruses isolated from patients in China, February to April 2013. *Euro Surveill,* 2013. 18(15): p. 20453.

[39] Liu, D., et al., Origin and diversity of novel avian influenza A H7N9 viruses causing human infection: phylogenetic, structural, and coalescent analyses. *Lancet,* 2013. 381(9881): p. 1926-32.

[40] Zhang, L., Z. Zhang, and Z. Weng, Rapid Reassortment of Internal Genes in Avian Influenza A(H7N9) Virus. *Clin Infect Dis,* 2013. 57(7): p. 1059-61.

[41] Wu, A., et al., Sequential reassortments underlie diverse influenza H7N9 genotypes in China. *Cell Host Microbe,* 2013. 14(4): p. 446-52.

[42] Cui, L., et al., Dynamic reassortments and genetic heterogeneity of the human-infecting influenza A (H7N9) virus. *Nat Commun,* 2014. 5: p. 3142.

[43] Wang, D., et al., Genetic tuning of the novel avian influenza A(H7N9) virus during interspecies transmission, China, 2013. *Euro Surveill,* 2014. 19(25): p. pii=20836.

[44] Horimoto, T. and Y. Kawaoka, Reverse genetics provides direct evidence for a correlation of hemagglutinin cleavability and virulence of an avian influenza A virus. *J Virol,* 1994. 68(5): p. 3120-8.

[45] Herfst, S., et al., Airborne transmission of influenza A/H5N1 virus between ferrets. *Science,* 2012. 336(6088): p. 1534-41.

[46] Matrosovich, M., et al., The surface glycoproteins of H5 influenza viruses isolated from humans, chickens, and wild aquatic birds have distinguishable properties. *J Virol,* 1999. 73(2): p. 1146-55.

[47] Guo, Y.J., et al., Characterization of the pathogenicity of members of the newly established H9N2 influenza virus lineages in Asia. *Virology,* 2000. 267(2): p. 279-88.

[48] Munier, S., et al., A genetically engineered waterfowl influenza virus with a deletion in the stalk of the neuraminidase has increased virulence for chickens. *J Virol,* 2010. 84(2): p. 940-52.

[49] Shi, W.F., et al., Genetic analysis of four porcine avian influenza viruses isolated from Shandong, China. *Arch Virol,* 2008. 153(1): p. 211-7.

[50] Spackman, E., et al., Sequence analysis of recent H7 avian influenza viruses associated with three different outbreaks in commercial poultry in the United States. *J Virol,* 2003. 77(24): p. 13399-402.

[51] Gabriel, G., A. Herwig, and H.D. Klenk, Interaction of polymerase subunit PB2 and NP with importin alpha1 is a determinant of host range of influenza A virus. *PLoS Pathog,* 2008. 4(2): p. e11.

[52] Matrosovich, M., J. Stech, and H.D. Klenk, Influenza receptors, polymerase and host range. *Rev Sci Tech,* 2009. 28(1): p. 203-17.

[53] Colman, P.M., Structural basis of antigenic variation: studies of influenza virus neuraminidase. *Immunol Cell Biol,* 1992. 70 (Pt 3): p. 209-14.

[54] Kiso, M., et al., Effect of an asparagine-to-serine mutation at position 294 in neuraminidase on the pathogenicity of highly pathogenic H5N1 influenza A virus. *J Virol,* 2011. 85(10): p. 4667-72.

[55] Yen, H.L., et al., Neuraminidase inhibitor-resistant influenza viruses may differ substantially in fitness and transmissibility. *Antimicrob Agents Chemother,* 2005. 49(10): p. 4075-84.

[56] Hu, Y.W., et al., Association between adverse clinical outcome in human disease caused by novel influenza A H7N9 virus and sustained viral shedding and emergence of antiviral resistance. *Lancet,* 2013. 381(9885): p. 2273-2279.

[57] Hay, A.J., et al., The molecular basis of the specific anti-influenza action of amantadine. *EMBO J,* 1985. 4(11): p. 3021-4.

[58] Xu, J., et al., Reducing exposure to avian influenza H7N9. *Lancet,* 2013. 381(9880): p. 1815-6.

[59] Horby, P., H7N9 is a virus worth worrying about. *Nature,* 2013. 496(7446): p. 399.

[60] Lazer, D., et al., Big data. The parable of Google Flu: traps in big data analysis. *Science,* 2014. 343(6176): p. 1203-5.

[61] Barclay, E., Predicting the next pandemic. *Lancet,* 2008. 372(9643): p. 1025-6.

[62] Soares Magalhaes, R.J., et al., Associations between attributes of live poultry trade and HPAI H5N1 outbreaks: a descriptive and network analysis study in northern Vietnam. *BMC Vet Res,* 2010. 6: p. 10.

[63] van den Berg, T., The role of the legal and illegal trade of live birds and avian products in the spread of avian influenza. *Rev Sci Tech,* 2009. 28(1): p. 93-111.

[64] Gong, C., et al., PageRank tracker: from ranking to tracking. *IEEE Trans Cybern,* 2014. 44(6): p. 882-93.

[65] Dellavalle, R.P., et al., Refining dermatology journal impact factors using PageRank. *J Am Acad Dermatol,* 2007. 57(1): p. 116-9.

[66] Lu, S., et al., [Investigating geographical spread of the human infection with avian influenza A (H7N9)virus by online knowledge analysis of the live bird trade with a distributed focused crawler]. *Zhonghua Liu Xing Bing Xue Za Zhi,* 2014. 35(3): p. 228-30.

[67] Chen, C., et al., Silent geographical spread of the H7N9 virus by online knowledge analysis of the live bird trade with a distributed focused crawler. *Emerging Microbes & Infections,* 2013. 2: p. e89.

[68] Vijaykrishna, D., et al., Evolutionary dynamics and emergence of panzootic H5N1 influenza viruses. *Plos Pathogens,* 2008. 4(9).

[69] Sun, Y., et al., Genotypic evolution and antigenic drift of H9N2 influenza viruses in China from 1994 to 2008. *Vet Microbiol,* 2010. 146(3-4): p. 215-25.

[70] Zhao, G., et al., Molecular evolution of the H6 subtype influenza A viruses from poultry in eastern China from 2002 to 2010. *Virol J,* 2011. 8: p. 470.

[71] Wang, G., et al., H6 influenza viruses pose a potential threat to human health. *J Virol,* 2014. 88(8): p. 3953-64.

[72] Shi, W., et al., Origin and molecular characterization of the human-infecting H6N1 influenza virus in Taiwan. *Protein Cell,* 2013. 4(11): p. 846-53.

[73] Chen, H., et al., Clinical and epidemiological characteristics of a fatal case of avian influenza A H10N8 virus infection: a descriptive study. *Lancet,* 2014. 383(9918): p. 714-21.

[74] Shi, W., et al., Phylogenetics of varied subtypes of avian influenza viruses in China: potential threat to humans. *Protein Cell,* 2014. 5(4): p. 253-7.

[75] Lu, J., et al., Continuing Reassortment Leads to the Genetic Diversity of Influenza Virus H7N9 in Guangdong, China. *J Virol,* 2014. 88(15): p. 8297-8306.

[76] Ozaki, H., et al., Changing patterns of h6 influenza viruses in Hong Kong poultry markets. *Influenza Res Treat,* 2011. 2011: p. 702092.

[77] Huang, K., et al., Establishment and lineage replacement of H6 influenza viruses in domestic ducks in southern China. *J Virol,* 2012. 86(11): p. 6075-83.

[78] Cheung, C.L., et al., Establishment of influenza A virus (H6N1) in minor poultry species in southern China. *J Virol,* 2007. 81(19): p. 10402-12.

[79] Chin, P.S., et al., Molecular evolution of H6 influenza viruses from poultry in Southeastern China: prevalence of H6N1 influenza viruses possessing seven A/Hong Kong/156/97 (H5N1)-like genes in poultry. *J Virol,* 2002. 76(2): p. 507-16.

[80] Yuan, J., et al., Origin and molecular characteristics of a novel 2013 avian influenza A(H6N1) virus causing human infection in Taiwan. *Clin Infect Dis,* 2013. 57(9): p. 1367-8.

[81] Guan, Y., et al., H5N1: How to track a flu virus. *Nature,* 2012. 483(7391): p. 535-6.

[82] Liu, D., W. Shi, and G.F. Gao, Poultry carrying H9N2 act as incubators for novel human avian influenza viruses. *Lancet,* 2014. 383(9920): p. 869.

[83] Liu, D. and G.F. Gao, The new emerging H7N9 influenza virus indicates poultry as new. *Sci China Life Sci,* 2014.

[84] Gao, G.F., Influenza and the live poultry trade. *Science,* 2014. 344(6181): p. 235.

In: Influenza and RNA Viruses
Editor: R. H. Bishop, pp. 79-89

ISBN: 978-1-63321-799-7

Chapter 4

ADAPTATION OF MATRIX PROTEIN 1 OF INFLUENZA A VIRUS TO CHANGE IN GLOBAL TEMPERATURE

Shaomin Yan and Guang Wu*
State Key Laboratory of Non-food Biomass Enzyme Technology,
National Engineering Research Center for Non-food Biorefinery,
Guangxi Biomass Industrialization Engineering Institute,
Guangxi Key Laboratory of Biorefinery, Guangxi Academy of Sciences,
Nanning, Guangxi, China

Abstract

Currently global temperature change is a major aspect of climate changes so it is important to study how proteins of influenza A viruses adapt to temperature change because the understanding of this adaptation would help us to deal with influenza epidemics and pandemics. In order to get a whole picture on the adaptation in influenza A virus, we studied the adaptation of matrix protein 1 (M1) from influenza A virus to global temperature change. 2116 M1 proteins sampled from 1918 to October 2012 were converted by predictable portion and compared with the temperature changes (HadCRUT3v and CRUTEM4v data sets) in a 5° by 5° grid-box basis. Still, point-to-point comparisons were made from 1959 to 1998 in all and different species. The results showed that changes in temperatures and predictable portion of M1 proteins had similar trends during

* E-mail address: hongguanglishibahao@yahoo.com; Tel: +86 771 2503 940; Fax: +86 771 2503 940; Address: 98 Daling Road, Nanning, Guangxi, 530007, China (Corresponding Author).

the period, highlighting impact of climate changes on influenza A viruses evolution.

Keywords: Adaptation, climate change, global temperature, influenza A virus, matrix protein 1

Introduction

Epidemics and pandemics of influenza impose severe challenges to public health [1]. These challenges are related to each aspect of public health [2], and have special implication to Southeast Asia, where is the source of many outbreaks due to the fact that swine, birds and humans live nearly, which provides good opportunity for viral mixing and mutating [3]. It is understandable that migrations of birds and large-scale growth of domestic animals make the people living in Southeast Asia susceptible to influenza virus. However, a new factor now should be added into our consideration in public health, that is, climate change, especially temperature change, over years, because temperature change can influence the habit and routes of migrations of birds and living conditions for domestic animals, and consequently influenza viruses would be affected alike [4].

Nevertheless, influenza viruses evolve to adapt changes in environments, and such adaptation goes through mutations in their proteins [5]. However, this is the key point leading to epidemics and pandemics of influenza because unpredictable mutations neutralize vaccines and anti-virus drugs. Technically it is almost impossible to predict mutations in influenza viruses because mutations can be attributed to various short-term as well as long-term factors, which are still very difficult to determine one by one. Yet, the change in global temperature is certainly a long-term factor, which not only impacts mutations in influenza viruses, but also provides us a clue to trace mutations in reference to adaptation.

Along this line of research thought, we have studied adaptation with respect to global temperature in seven of eleven proteins of influenza A viruses including hemagglutinin, neuraminidase, nucleoprotein, polymerase acidic protein, polymerase basic proteins 1 and 2, and matrix protein 2 [6-11]. It is necessary to study each protein from influenza A virus in order to get a whole picture.

The matrix protein 1 (M1) of influenza A virus regulates the bi-directional transport of ribonucleoprotein into and out of the nucleus, and plays important roles in various steps of virus replication, assembly and budding [12-14]. M1 can bind to the cytoplasmic tails of HA and NA to form the interior structure of the emerging virion. M1 can serve as a docking site for the recruitment of the viral

RNPs, and may mediate the recruitment of M2 to the site of virus budding [15]. Also, in animal model a live attenuated H1N1 M1 mutant can provide broad cross-protection against influenza A viruses [16]. Therefore it is important to study M1's adaptation with respect to changes in global temperature, which is designed as the aim of this study.

Materials and Methods

Temperature Data

The global temperature anomalies from 1850 to October 2012, whose anomaly was based on the period 1961-1990, were obtained from HadCRUT3v [17, 18]. The local temperature from 1959 to 1998 was based on 0.5 by 0.5° latitude and longitude grid-box basis cross globe [19].

M1 Data

22061 full-length M1 sequences of influenza A viruses sampled from 1918 to October 2012 were obtained from the Influenza Research Database [20]. After being removed duplicate sequences, 2158 M1 proteins were actually used in this study.

M1 Evolution

The trend of temperature is temperature along the time course, and equally we need present M1 evolution as a trend along the time course. In this way, we can compare whether both trends run forwards similar, or opposite, or directionless direction. In order to keep consistent with our previous studies [6-11], we use the amino-acid pair predictability as an indicator to present M1 evolution [21-25].

For example, an M1 protein (accession number CY084556) from A/swine/Hong Kong/33/1977(H1N1) is composed of 252 amino acids, which are counted as 251 adjacent amino-acid pairs. There are 17 glutamic acids "E" and 26 alanines "A" in this M1: if permutation can predict the appearance of amino-acid pair EA, it would appear twice ($17/252 \times 26/251 \times 251 = 1.75$), and it does appear twice so its appearance is predictable. By contrast, there are 26 leucines "L" and 13 lysines "K" in this protein: if permutation can predict the appearance of amino-acid pair LK, it would appear once (26/252×13/251×251 = 1.34), however, it appears 4 times in realty so its appearance is unpredictable.

In this way, we classified all amino-acid pairs in this M1 protein as predictable and unpredictable portions, which are 26.29% and 73.71%. For another M1 protein (accession number CY084596) from A/swine/Hong Kong/39/1977(H1N1), it has only one amino acid at position 192 different from CY084556 M1 protein, but its predictable and unpredictable portions are 25.5% and 74.5%. Therefore each M1 protein has its own predictable/unpredictable portion, and 2158 M1 proteins were converted into 2158 different predictable/unpredictable portions. As each M1 was sample in certain place in certain year, its predictable/unpredictable portion at sampling year and location can correspond to the temperature recorded at the same time and location, by which we observed their trend along the time course, and even more exactly made point-to-point comparisons at the same location.

Results and Discussion

Four human influenza pandemics have been recorded in 1918, 1957, 1968 and 2009, and many reasons for inducing the emergence of deadly virus variants have been explored. Among them is La Niña conditions in the equatorial Pacific and changes in the phase of the El Niño-Southern oscillation [26].

These climate changes can alter natural reservoir of influenza A viruses, such as migration pattern, stopover time, fitness and interspecies mixing of birds, which demonstrates the effect of climate changes on influenza A viruses. Naturally, changes in global temperature would lay the foundation for unpredictable mutations in influenza A viruses under other climate changes, because changes in global temperature may influence influenza A viruses when two trends are almost parallel or opposite.

Figure 1 shows the progressive increase in global temperature (upper panel), and the progressive increase in M1 evolution in terms of predictable portion (lower panel) from 1918 to 2012. Because only a few data are available prior to 1959, our analysis was focused on the data between 1959 and 2012 (Figure 2). The regression was applied to general trends resulting in different slopes of regressed lines. First, the both trends represented as regressed lines have a similar direction, which suggests that changes in global temperature affect M1 evolution otherwise M1 evolution would be directionless. Second, the different slopes imply different speeds regarding changes in global temperature and M1 evolution, which

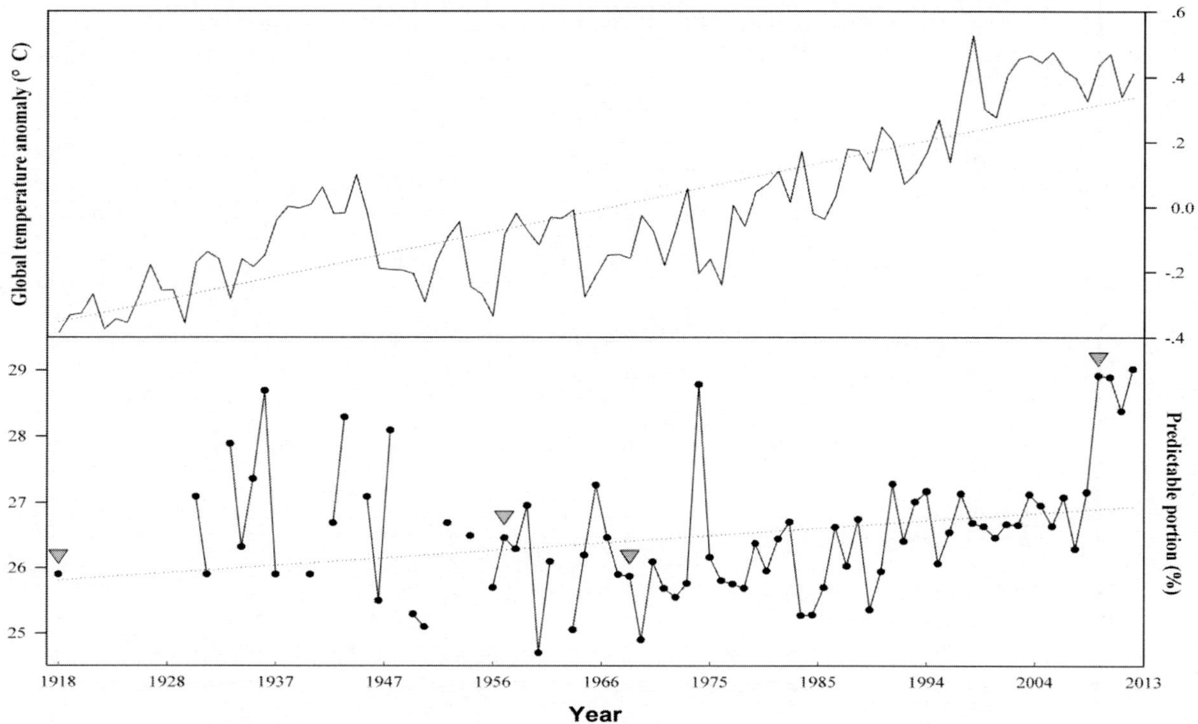

Figure 1. Changes in global temperature and M1 proteins of influenza A viruses from 1918 to 2012 (n = 2158). The dotted lines were regressed lines. The circles represented the mean predictable portion of all M1 proteins at a given year. The down triangles indicated four influenza pandemics occurred.

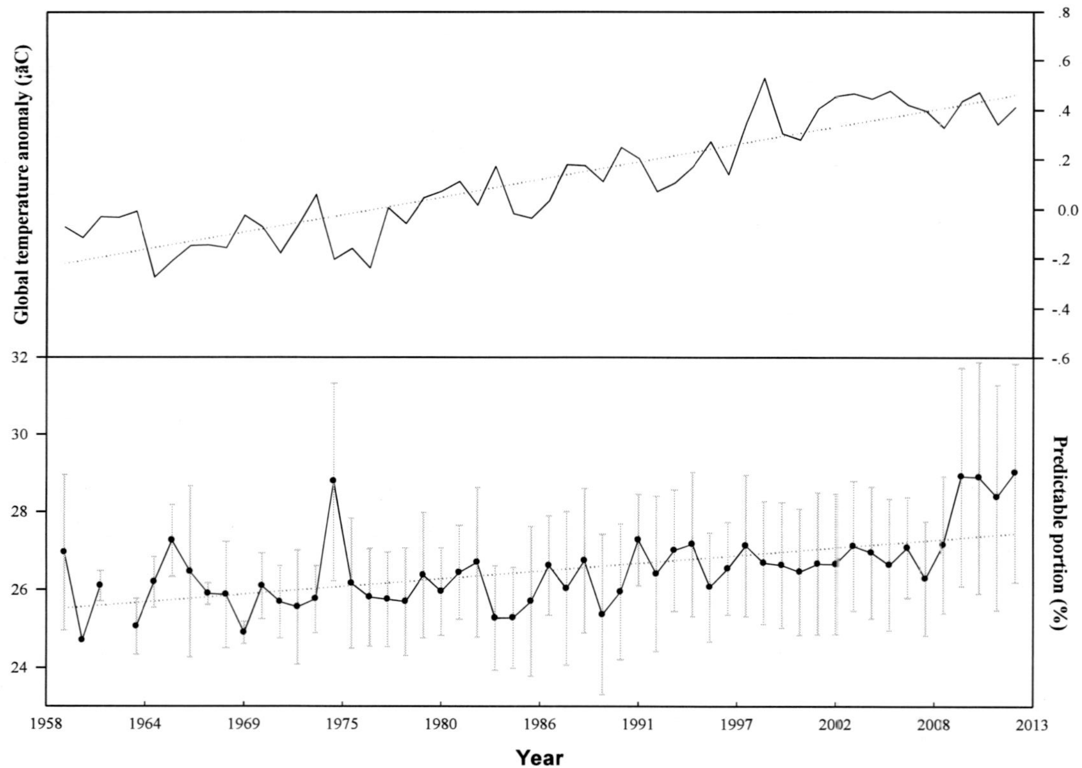

Figure 2. Changes in global temperature and M1 proteins of influenza A viruses from 1959 to 2012 (n = 2116). The dotted lines were regressed lines. The circles with gray bars indicated the mean ± SD of predictable portion calculated from all M1 proteins at a given year.

are expected because M1 adaptation should be slower than changes in global temperature. Third, we could not exclude the possibility that the different slopes are due to the unbalance of data because M1 data in Figures 1 and 2 are averaged for each year. For example, there are only 3 M1 proteins in 1959, but there are 316 M1 proteins in 2009; meanwhile the similar situation would be expected in collection of temperature data because more and more metrological stations are built.

Thereafter, we developed our observation through location-to-location along the time course.

For example, the AY210032 M1 protein was sampled in 1959 at Ohio, USA, whose latitude and longitude are 40.37° and –82.67° according to Get Lat Lon [27], where the average yearly temperature was 10.55°C in 1959 according to the 0.5° by 0.5° latitude and longitude grid-box basis cross globe [17].

Figure 3 displays 291 location-to-location relationships between temperature and M1 evolution in terms of the predictable portion from 1959 to 1998, where it can be seen that their regressions have similar slopes, which furthermore confirm

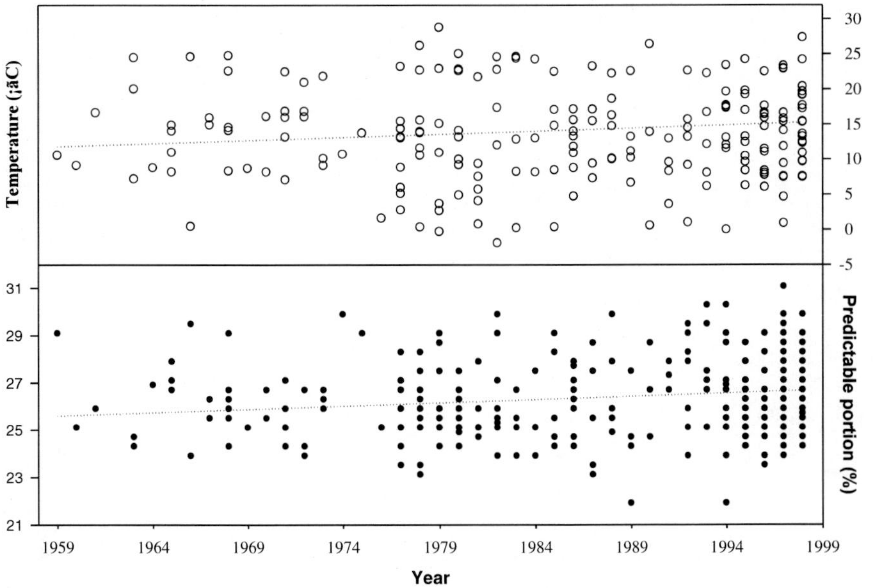

Figure 3. Location-to-location temperature versus M1 proteins (n = 291) from 1959 to 1998. Each point presented a local temperature (°C) at the given year (upper panel), corresponding to the place where a M1 protein was sampled (lower panel). The dotted lines were regressed lines.

what shown in Figures 1 and 2, say, trends for global temperature and M1 evolution move forwards to a similar direction over the last half a century.

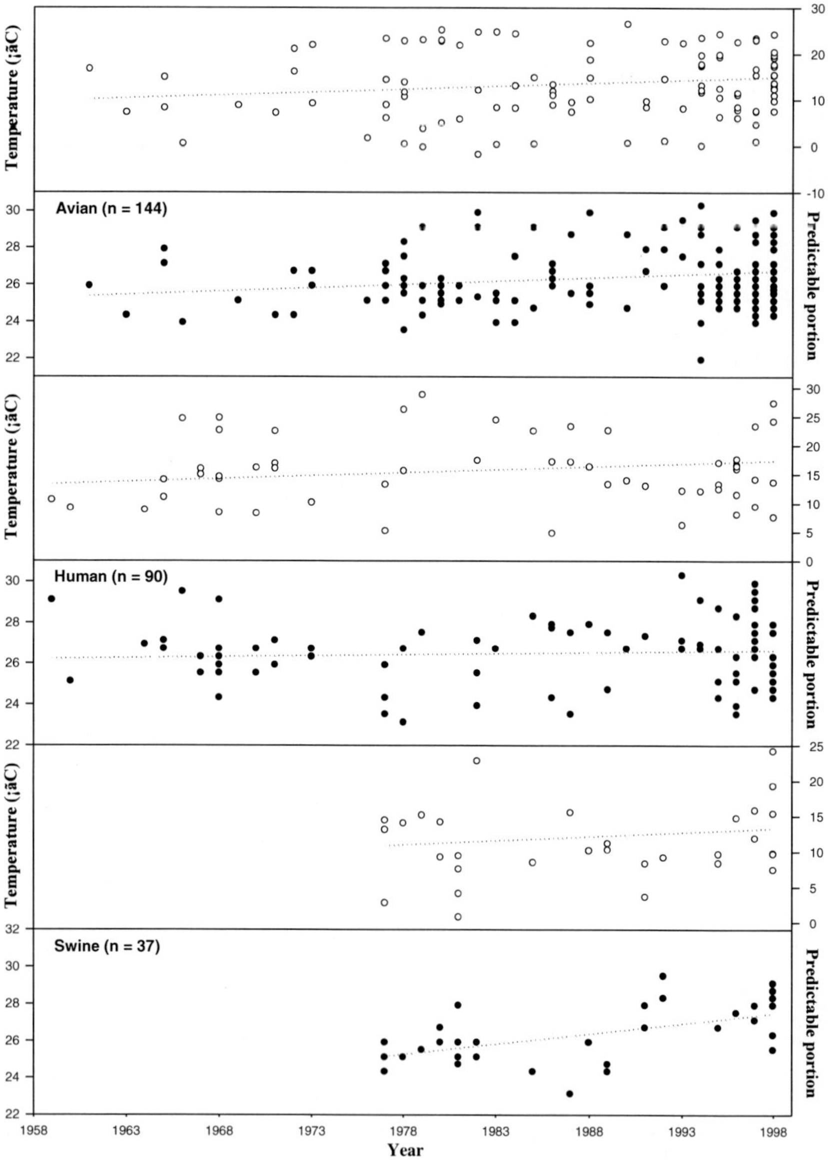

Figure 4. Location-to-location temperature (°C) versus M1 proteins sampled from different species. The dotted lines were regressed lines.

Individual influenza A virus must replicate in a specific host, which depends on many factors, including viral proteins, host system and environmental conditions [28]. Thus we advanced our knowledge through the location-to-location relationship between temperature and species, where M1 proteins were sampled. Figure 4 shows the trends of M1 evolution in three major species (avian, human and swine) with respect to the temperature, where we can see the similar trends between temperature and M1 evolution regarding these species, indicating that adaptation of influenza A viruses to temperature change can be found in different species.

The evolution of influenza A viruses in their reservoir hosts and consequently their genetic changes can form novel viruses into humans, which may result in seasonal epidemics or even pandemics [29].

Conclusion

Using predictable portion of amino acid pairs as an indicator, we analyzed matrix protein 1 of influenza A viruses. The results showed that changes in temperatures and predictable portion of M1 proteins had similar trends from 1918 to 2012. Influenza A viruses rapidly evolve to adapt their living environment and the current results are consistent with those of our previous ones, demonstrating the persistent impact of temperature change on the evolution of viral proteins.

Acknowledgments

This study was partly supported by Guangxi Science Foundation (2013GXNSDA019007 and 1347004-1) and Building of Guangxi Talent Highland.

References

[1] Morse SS, Mazet JA, Woolhouse M, Parrish CR, Carroll D, Karesh WB, Zambrana-Torrelio C, Lipkin WI, Daszak P. Prediction and prevention of the next pandemic zoonosis. *Lancet* 2012;380:1956-1965.

[2] Karesh WB, Dobson A, Lloyd-Smith JO, Lubroth J, Dixon MA, Bennett M, Aldrich S, Harrington T, Formenty P, Loh EH, Machalaba CC, Thomas MJ, Heymann DL. Ecology of zoonoses: natural and unnatural histories. *Lancet* 2012;380:1936-1945.

[3] Shao H. The evolution of influenza viruses. *Health* 2012;4(Special Issue):1000-1005.

[4] Brown VL, Drake JM, Stallknecht DE, Brown JD, Pedersen K, Rohani P. Dissecting a wildlife disease hotspot: the impact of multiple host species, environmental transmission and seasonality in migration, breeding and mortality. *J. R. Soc. Interface* 2013;10:20120804.

[5] Medina RA, García-Sastre A. Influenza A viruses: new research developments. *Nat. Rev. Microbiol.* 2011;9:590-603.

[6] Yan S, Wu G. What these trends suggest? *Am. J. Appl. Sci.* 2009;6:1116-1121.

[7] Yan S, Wu G. Trends in global warming and evolution of matrix protein 2 family from influenza A virus. *Interdiscip Sci. Comput Life Sci* 2009;1:272-279.

[8] Yan S, Wu G. Trends in global warming and evolution of polymerase basic protein 2 family from influenza A virus. *J. Biomed. Sci. Eng* 2009;2:458-464.

[9] Yan SM, Zuo WP, Zhu QX, Huang YY, Pan LX, Wu G. Trends in global warming and evolution of neuraminidases from influenza A viruses since 1918. *Guangxi Sci* 2010;17:80-84.

[10] Yan S, Wu G. Trends in global warming and evolution of nucleoproteins from influenza A viruses since 1918.*Transbound Emerg. Dis.* 2010;57:404-413.

[11] Yan S, Wu G. Adaptation in polymerase basic protein 1 family from influenza A virus to climate change. *Health* 2012;4:968-973.

[12] Barman S, Ali A, Hui EK, Adhikary L, Nayak DP. Transport of viral proteins to the apical membranes and interaction of matrix protein with glycoproteins in the assembly of influenza viruses. *Virus Res.* 2001;77:61-69.

[13] Boulo S, Akarsu H, Ruigrok RW, Baudin F. Nuclear traffic of influenza virus proteins and ribonucleoprotein complexes. *Virus Res.* 2007;124:12-21.

[14] Huang S, Chen J, Wang H, Sun B, Wang H, Zhang Z, et al. Influenza A virus matrix protein 1 interacts with hTFIIIC102-s, a short isoform of the polypeptide 3 subunit of human general transcription factor IIIC. *Arch Virol* 2009;154:1101-1010.

[15] Rossman JS, Lamb RA. Influenza virus assembly and budding. *Virology* 2011;411:229-236.

[16] Xie H, Liu TM, Lu X, Wu Z, Belser JA, Katz JM, Tumpey TM, Ye Z. A live attenuated H1N1 M1 mutant provides broad cross-protection against

influenza A viruses, including highly pathogenic A/Vietnam/1203/2004, in mice. *J. Infect. Dis.* 2009;200:1874-1883.

[17] Jones P, Harpham C, Salmon M. *Climatic Research Unit.* 2013. Available at: http://www.cru.uea.ac.uk/cru/data/temperature/.

[18] Rayner NA, Brohan P, Parker DE, Folland CK, Kennedy JJ, Vanicek M, Ansell T, Tett SFB. Improved analyses of changes and uncertainties in marine temperature measured in situ since the mid nineteenth century: The HadSST2 dataset. *J. Clim.* 2006;19:446-469.

[19] New M, Hulme M, Jones P. Representing twentieth-century space-time climate variability. Part II: Development of 1901-96 monthly grids of terrestrial surface climate. *J. Clim.* 2000;13:2217-2238.

[20] Squires RB, Noronha J, Hunt V, García-Sastre A, Macken C, Baumgarth N, Suarez D, Pickett BE, Zhang Y, Larsen CN, Ramsey A, Zhou L, Zaremba S, Kumar S, Deitrich J, Klem E, Scheuermann RH. Influenza research database: an integrated bioinformatics resource for influenza research and surveillance. *Influenza Other Respi. Viruses* 2012;6:404-416.

[21] Wu G, Yan SM. Randomness in the primary structure of protein: methods and implications. *Mol Biol Today* 2002;3:55-69.

[22] Wu G, Yan S. Fate of influenza A virus proteins. *Protein Pept. Lett.* 2006;13:377-384.

[23] Wu G, Yan S. Mutation trend of hemagglutinin of influenza A virus: a review from computational mutation viewpoint. *Acta Pharmacol. Sin.* 2006;27:513-526.

[24] Wu G, Yan S. *Lecture notes on computational mutation.* New York: Nova Science Publishers; 2008.

[25] Yan SM, Wu G. Fitting of global temperature change from 1850 to 2009 using random walk. *Guangxi. Sci.* 2010;17:148-150.

[26] Shaman J, Lipsitch M. The El Nino-Southern Oscillation (ENSO)-pandemic Influenza connection: coincident or causal? *Proc. Natl. Acad. Sci. U S A* 2013;110 (Suppl 1): 3689-3691.

[27] Willison S. *Get Lat Lon.* 2013. Available at: http://www.getlatlon.com/.

[28] Yassine HM, Lee CW, Gourapura R, Saif YM. Interspecies and intraspecies transmission of influenza A viruses: viral, host and environmental factors. *Anim. Health Res. Rev.* 2010;11:53-72.

[29] Taubenberger JK, Kash JC. Influenza virus evolution, host adaptation, and pandemic formation. *Cell Host Microbe* 2010;7:440-451.

In: Influenza and RNA Viruses
Editor: R. H. Bishop, pp. 91-110

ISBN: 978-1-63321-799-7

Chapter 5

APPLICATION OF CELL SURFACE ENGINEERED YEAST FOR THE DEVELOPMENT OF DRUGS AGAINST INFLUENZA VIRUS INFECTION

***Junki Yamada*[1], *Natsuko Miura*[1,2], *Tomohiro Shigemori*[1], *Kouichi Kuroda*[1] *and Mitsuyoshi Ueda*[1]**

[1]Division of Applied Life Sciences, Graduate School of Agriculture, Kyoto University, Kyoto, Japan

[2]Frontier Research Core for Life Science, University of Toyama, Toyama, Japan

Abstract

Influenza A viruses, which are members of the orthomyxovirus family, cause epidemics and pandemics throughout the world. Recently, a novel swine-origin H1N1 influenza virus emerged, and human-to-human transmission of this virus led to the declaration of a pandemic by the World Health Organization (WHO) in 2009.

In addition, highly pathogenic H5N1 avian influenza viruses were detected in Hong Kong in 1997. Although the H5N1 viruses had not caused a pandemic until now, they could cause a pandemic at any time because mutations frequently occur in influenza viruses. Various approaches have been used to neutralize influenza viruses, such as anti-influenza virus drugs and vaccines.

Their main targets are hemagglutinin (HA) and neuraminidase (NA), two membrane proteins on the influenza virus that are major determinants of pathogenicity. It has been reported that HA and NA mutations occur frequently, which makes treating of influenza virus infections difficult. Although we can promptly analyze the DNA sequences of HA and NA genes derived from mutant viruses by using next-generation DNA sequencing technology, the DNA sequence does not provide functional information for the proteins encoded by the mutant DNAs. Such protein analyses are difficult because purification of the recombinant proteins includes burdensome steps. Here, we introduce a new approach to solve this problem using a yeast cell surface engineering system. Using this system, it is possible to easily construct a comprehensive mutant protein library that is displayed on the yeast cell surface using the sequence of individual mutant DNAs, because the various inconvenient and troublesome steps of protein preparations can be avoided. In addition, it can be used to quickly evaluate whether the presently available drugs, such as oseltamivir and zanamivir, could be effective against the mutant proteins. HA- and NA-displaying yeasts can be targets for screening novel inhibitors in an available chemical library. In addition, the mutant proteins encoded by mutations that may occur in the future can be predictably prepared. We review the advantages of these approaches for influenza therapy.

Introduction

Influenza virus infection is a serious public health concern, and another influenza pandemic could occur at any time. Influenza viruses are classified as A, B, and C types based on the present nucleoproteins [1]. Types A and B cause pandemics. Type A viruses have membrane proteins, such as hemagglutinin (HA) and neuraminidase (NA), which have 16 and 9 subtypes, respectively [2, 3]. These subtypes are defined by their interactions with antibodies, and all viruses of the same subtype are neutralized by a specific antibody. Influenza viruses have various combinations of HA and NA proteins, and can infect not only swine and poultry but also humans [4]. Influenza virus binds to sialic acids on the host cell surface, and is then taken into the cell by endocytosis. The membrane of the influenza virus becomes fused with the host cell membrane through HA. The virus then releases its RNAs into the cytosol of the host cell. The RNAs are translated in the host cell, and the translated proteins are packaged by the host lipid bilayer membrane. Because the packaged virus particle is released by exocytosis, but binds to sialic acid on the host cell surface, cleavage of sialic acid by NA is required for complete release of the influenza virus (Figure 1) [5]. Influenza viruses can escape detection by the host immune system because they continuously evolve by antigenic drift and shift. "Antigenic drift" is a moderate evolution caused by the occurrence of frequent mutations. In the influenza virus, it involves the generation of point mutations in HA and NA during viral replication [6].These mutations allow the virus to evade host neutralizing antibodies and to spread more effectively [7]. "Antigenic shift" is the replacement of the existing HA and NA subtypes with new subtypes [8]. Genetic reassortment, which is caused by co-circulation of different influenza subtypes, contributes to antigenic shift [9]. This generates new influenza viruses that humans have never encountered before. These influenza viruses have caused several pandemics, including the Spanish influenza (H1N1), Asian influenza (H2N2), Hong Kong influenza (H3N2), and Russian influenza (H1N1) [10]. In 1997, human infection by the highly pathogenic H5N1 avian influenza viruses was confirmed in Hong Kong [11]. Although H5N1 viruses lack the ability to transmit from human to human, mutant H5N1 viruses that newly acquire human-to-human infectious ability could emerge at any time.

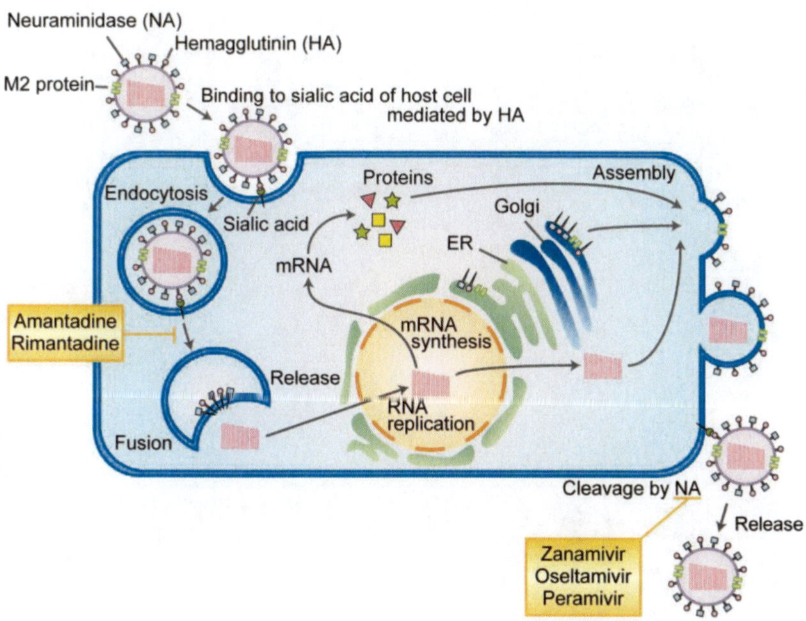

Figure 1. Life cycle of the influenza virus [10]. In this illustration, several commercial inhibitors are shown.

In this chapter, the approaches used to treat the disease caused by influenza virus infection are examined, and we present novel methods to address the frequently mutated influenza viruses using yeast cell surface engineering.

1. Antigenic Proteins of Influenza Virus

HA is a homotrimeric membrane glycoprotein. Each monomer of HA has a core α helix and an active head domain that is involved in the binding to sialic acid [12, 13]. The monomer is translated as a precursor called HA0 (Figure 2A) [14]. Cleavage of HA0 generates the active form, which is composed of the C terminus of HA1 and the N terminus of HA2 and is required for membrane fusion activity and infectivity (Figure 2B) [15].

At the beginning of infection, the virus binds to the host cell via sialic acid, which exists as different linkage types, such as α2-3 and α2-6, and then enters the host cells by endocytosis. An irreversible conformational change in HA that occurs at low pH exposes the N-terminal HA2 fusion peptide (Figure 2B), while preserving the structure of the HA1 receptor-binding domain (Figure 2B) [16].

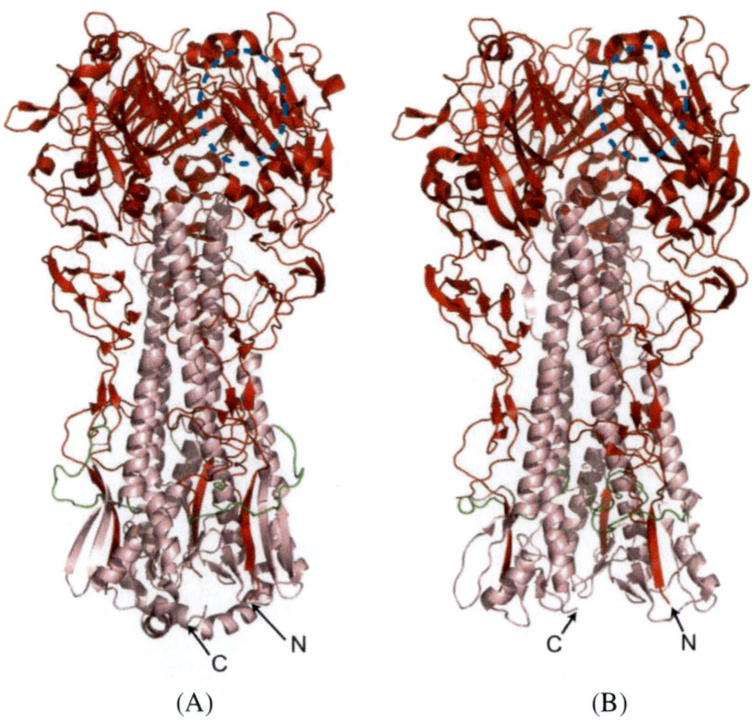

Figure 2. Crystal structures of (A) the precursor form of HA (HA0; PDB entry: 1RD8 [HP: http://www.rcsb.org/]) and (B) the active form of HA (PDB entry: 1RUZ). Red: HA1 (head domain), Light pink: HA2 (stem domain), Blue dot circle: receptor-binding domain, Green: fusion peptide, N: N-terminal position, C: C-terminal position.

Because the fusion peptide is nonpolar, it can insert into the target cell membrane [17]. The exact mechanism of influenza virus HA-host membrane fusion has not yet been clarified; however, some hypothetical mechanisms are presented in Figure 3 [18, 19].

NA exists as a mushroom-shaped projection on the surface of the influenza virus [5]. It has a head domain (Figure 4A) consisting of four subunits (Figure 4B) and a hydrophobic transmembrane region (stem domain). NA is an enzyme that aids in virus release from the host cell [5].

Although HA on the surface of the virion is required for invasion, it inhibits release of the newly-produced virus particle. NA cleaves the terminal sialic acid residues from the glycan structures on the surface of the infected cell. This enables the release of progeny viruses from the host cell, and their spread from the infected cell to uninfected surrounding cells [20].

The functional and quantitative balances of HA and NA are also important for virus replication [21].

2. Treatments for Influenza Virus Infection

Amantadine (Figure 5A) and its analogue rimantadine (Figure 5B) are antiviral chemical drugs used for the treatment of influenza A virus infection. These drugs inhibit the ion channel function of the M2 protein, which is important for virus replication due to its role of pH regulation inside the virus (Figure 1) [22, 23]. However, these drugs are not effective against influenza B virus because it does not possess an M2 protein. In addition, clinical use of these drugs has been

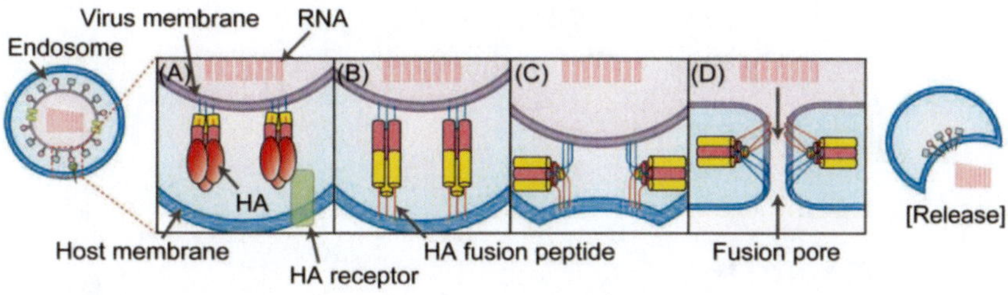

Figure 3. Hypothetical mechanisms for influenza virus membrane fusion through viral glycoproteins [18, 19]. (A) Virus membrane with HA molecules and the host membrane. (B) The conformational change induced at low pH allows insertion of the fusion peptide into the host membrane. (C) HA draws the membranes together. (D) Formation of the fusion pore leads to transfer of the viral genome.

limited because of their side effects due to their inhibitory activity against endogenous ion channel activity in patients [24] and the rapid emergence of viruses with mutated M2 proteins, that are resistant to these drugs [25].

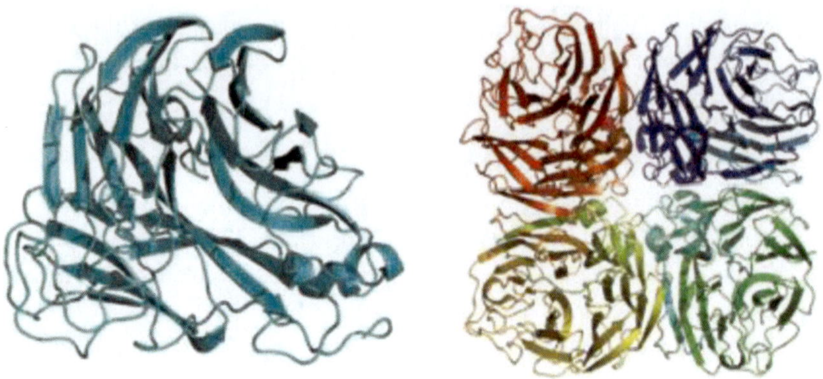

(A) (B)

Figure 4. Crystal structure of (A) the head domain of an NA monomer (PDB entry: 3TI6) and (B) the NA homotetramer (PDB entry: 2B8H).

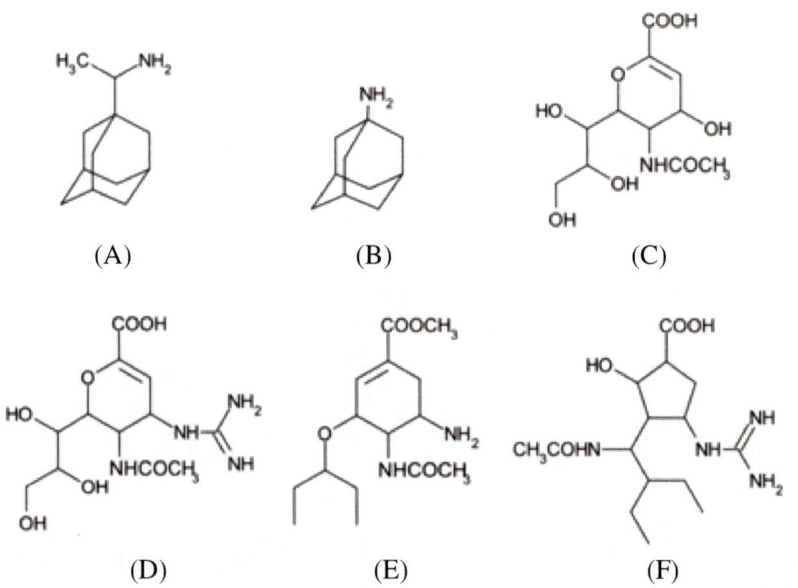

Figure 5. Structures of anti-influenza drugs. (A) amantadine, (B) rimantadine, (C) Neu5Ac2en, (D) zanamivir, (E) oseltamivir, and (F) peramivir.

HA is one of the main targets of anti-influenza drugs. The three main stages in the maturation of HA, cleavage of HA0, recognition of the host receptor, and the conformational change required for membrane fusion, each present a different target for inhibition by antiviral agents.

Inhibition of HA0 cleavage, which induces HA maturation and is essential for subsequent stages of infection [26], has been achieved by using peptidyl chloroalkyl ketone inhibitors of the protease furin [27].

Sialic acid-mimic peptides that function as HA inhibitors were obtained using phage display with a random pentadecapeptide library [28].

The pH-dependent, fusion-related conformational change is inhibited by *tert*-butyl hydroquinone (TBQH), which binds to a hydrophobic interface between the HA monomers [26]. At present, no HA inhibitors are marketed for clinical use.

HA is also the primary target for vaccine-induced neutralizing antibodies. However, HA escapes the host immune system by rapidly and continuously accumulating mutations. In addition, the current influenza vaccines induce neutralizing antibodies that recognize closely related subtypes, and cross-reactive antibodies are hardly produced by vaccination. Furthermore, predicting the subtype that could cause the next pandemics is almost impossible. Therefore, cross-reactive antibodies against HA subtypes were analyzed to determine the key factor that stimulates production of antibodies capable of neutralizing multiple HA subtypes [29]. The analysis revealed that a broadly neutralizing antibody recognized a highly conserved stem region of HA. This result suggests the possibility of designing a universal vaccine that induces the production of cross-reactive antibodies against influenza viruses.

By the way, because NA plays an important role in influenza virus expansion, as mentioned above, and has a highly conserved active site, selective inhibitors for NA have also been developed.

Early in the development of NA inhibitors, 2-deoxy-2,3-didehydro-2-deoxy-*N*-acetylneuraminic acid (Neu5Ac2en) was found to inhibit the activity of NA (Figure 5C). Neu5Ac2en binds to the active site of NA by mimicking the transition state during the enzymatic reaction. However, the inhibitory activity of Neu5Ac2en is not sufficient to prevent viral replication. To increase the binding ability toward NA active site, a computer-assisted approach based on the crystal structure of NA was used [30].

This study predicted energetically favorable substitutions in Neu5Ac2en by computational modeling and suggested that the replacement of the 4-hydroxy group with an amino or guanidinyl group would increase the binding affinity. Analysis of the crystal structures of 4-amino- and 4-guanidino-Neu5Ac2en revealed that the C4 amino group of 4-amino-Neu5Ac2en formed a salt bridge with Glu119 of NA (N2 numbering) [30], and that the interaction of the terminal guanidinyl nitrogens of 4-guanidino-Neu5Ac2en with both Glu119 and Glu227 (N2 numbering) resulted in tighter binding. 4-Guanidino-Neu5Ac2en is a more potent inhibitor of influenza virus replication than 4-amino-Neu5Ac2en. 4-Guanidino-Neu5Ac2en, which is also called zanamivir, became the first NA inhibitor approved for clinical use (Figure 5D). However, zanamivir is administered by inhalation because it has low oral bioavailability.

To address influenza pandemics or epidemics, it is necessary to develop orally available inhibitors because oral administration is more patient-friendly for both treatment and prophylaxis. Oseltamivir is an NA inhibitor designed to solve this problem [31] (Figure 5E). Analysis of the crystal structures of NA with Neu5Ac or its analogues revealed that the hydrophobic pocket in the active site of NA is a key to increasing the lipophilicity of these inhibitors, which is expected to improve their oral bioavailability. First, the dihydropyran ring was replaced with a carbocyclic ring to increase its chemical stability and make it easier to modify the structure. Second, the effect of replacing the glycerol moiety with lipophilic side chains was examined. Replacement with a 3-pentyl group produced the most suitable hydrophobic contact with the NA active site. Oseltamivir is administered as a prodrug, oseltamivir ethyl ester.

Then, the oseltamivir ethyl ester is absorbed and metabolized to active oseltamivir carboxylate. Its bioavailability is approximately 80% when orally administrated. Therefore, due to its ease of administration, oseltamivir replaced zanamivir as the NA inhibitor of choice.

However, NA mutants, such as H274Y (N2 numbering), have been reported to exhibit resistance to oseltamivir [32].

In addition, a zanamivir-resistant E119G variant (N2 numbering) of influenza virus has also been reported [33].

Peramivir (Figure 5F) was developed as a novel, orally active, potent, and selective inhibitor of influenza NA [34] based on the crystal structure of NA with Neu5Ac2en and α/β-6-acetyl-amino-3,6-dideoxy-D-glycero-altro-2-nonulofuranosonic acid [35]. The crystal structure of NA with Neu5Ac2en revealed four binding pockets in the active site: (1) an acidic pocket where the carboxylic acid of Neu5Ac2en interacts with three arginine residues by hydrogen bonding, (2) an acetamido binding pocket that forms a hydrophobic patch, (3) the glycerol binding pocket, and (4) the pocket occupied by the C4-hydroxyl of Neu5Ac2en. Peramivir has a cyclopentane ring as a scaffold, a guanidino group that interacts with the active site, like zanamivir, and an *n*-butyl side chain that forms hydrophobic contacts.Protein crystallography was used to detect the active isomer because there are several isomers of peramivir. Peramivir retains its inhibitory activity against the E119G NA mutant (N2 numbering), which is resistant to zanamivir [36] and has a slow off-rate compared to oseltamivir carboxylate and zanamivir [37].In clinical use, peramivir is administrated intravenously and is more promising for patients that are not able to take oral medicines by themselves.

As mentioned above, several approaches have been used to treat influenza virus infection. However, new mutant influenza viruses that cannot be treated with any current therapy may emerge at any time because mutations occur frequently. Therefore, it is necessary to develop a novel system to address the frequent mutations in influenza.

3. Applications of Yeast Cell Surface Engineering

3.1. Yeast Cell Surface Engineering

Yeast cell surface engineering is one of the most promising tools for addressing the problem of frequently mutated influenza viruses. The cell surface plays important roles not only in cell shape determination but also as a functional interface between the inside and outside of the cell. Cell surface engineering provides yeast with several advantages [38]. The yeast cell surface engineering system utilizes the genetic information of α-agglutinin. This protein contains a secretion signal at the N-terminus that targets it to the cell surface and a glycosylphosphatidylinositol (GPI) anchor-attachment signal at the C-terminus that is required for cell wall anchoring (Figure 6).

By constructing gene fusions containing these two signals, cell surface display of proteins can be achieved. In this system, after transcription and translation, precursor proteins are transported into the endoplasmic reticulum (ER) due to the presence of the N-terminal signal sequence.

In the ER, the GPI anchor-attachment signal is recognized and cleared. The proteins are then transported from the ER to the Golgi apparatus, and then to the plasma membrane via secretory vesicles.

Phosphatidylinositol-specific phospholipase C (PI-PLC) cleaves the protein as it is transiently anchored to the plasma membrane, and they finally bind covalently with glucan on the cell wall. It is easy to analyze the function of proteins using yeast cell surface engineering because some burdensome steps, including protein purification, can be avoided.

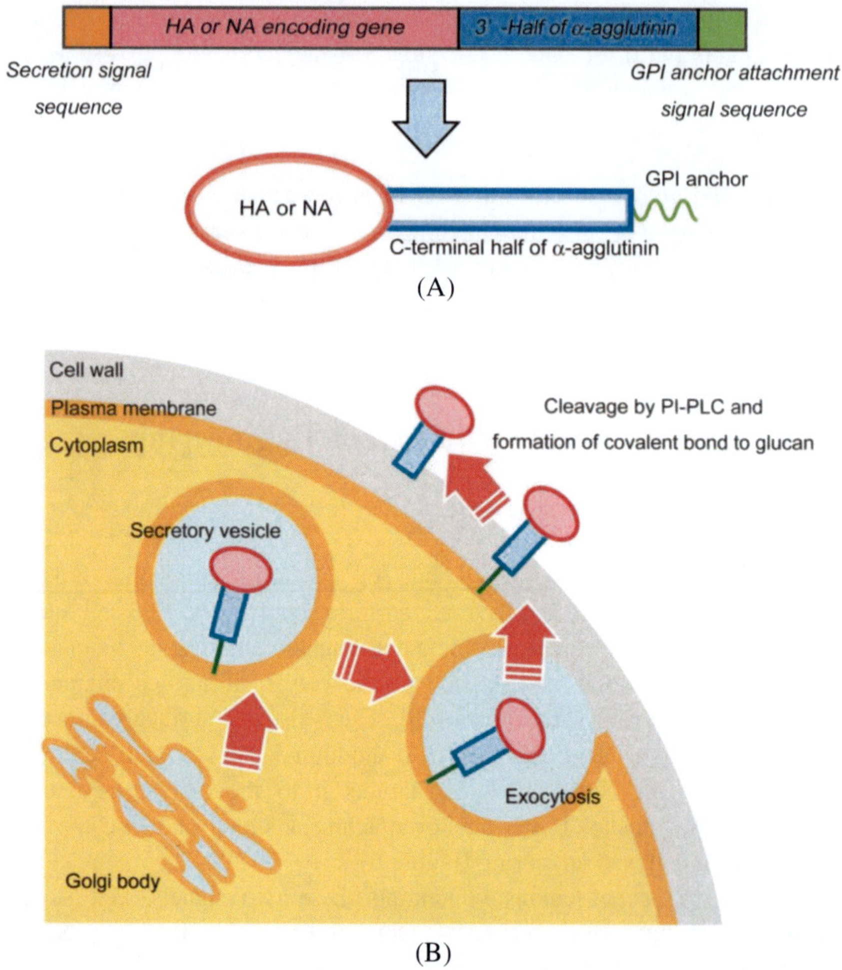

Figure 6. (A) Design of fusion genes for displaying HA or NA by cell surface engineering. (B) Mechanism of cell surface display of proteins via cell surface engineering [38, 39].

In addition, yeasts displaying a combinatorial protein library, following the introduction of DNAs with combinatorial mutations, allow us to analyze the features of these proteins in a high-throughput manner [39].

One of the advantages of cell surface engineering is that the altered proteins from mutant influenza viruses can be easily displayed by introducing the DNA sequences from these viruses.

3.2. Application of Yeast Cell Surface Engineering for the Treatment of Influenza Infection

Yeast can function as a host for enzyme production and as a carrier for enzyme immobilization (Figure 7). Therefore, yeast displaying the head domain of NA (HNA) without the transmembrane and stem regions could be used as a platform for inhibitor screening [40]. The wild type and the H274Y mutant HNA (N2 numbering), which exhibits resistance to oseltamivir, were successfully displayed on the yeast cell surface. Their activities could be detected easily without purification. The inhibition properties and IC_{50} values of oseltamivir carboxylate and zanamivir against these two HNAs were consistent with those of the previous report (Figure 8).

In addition, the displayed H274Y HNA was stable at 37 °C even though the thermal stability of the H274Y HNA mutant was reported to be reduced.

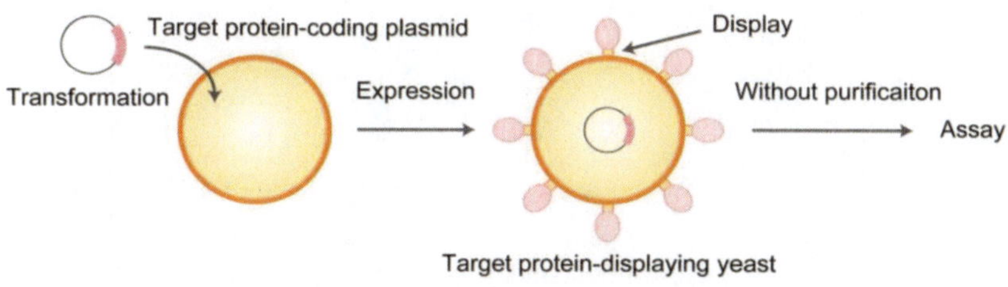

Figure 7. Advantages of using yeast cell surface engineering as a host for enzyme production and a carrier for displaying enzymes and mutant enzymes.

This system can be utilized for screening chemical libraries to obtain inhibitors of HA and NA mutants. It is necessary to screen large numbers of variants in a library to determine what binds to the proteins of interest. Computational design would enable us to predict specific interactions between test molecules and target proteins and to obtain high-affinity binders [41].

High-affinity binders were obtained by combining a computational method with yeast cell surface engineering [38, 42]. In this study, the proteins were designed to bind to the highly conserved stem region of HA, which is recognized by the cross-reactive antibody, and was displayed on the yeast cell surface with a c-Myc tag that is recognized by the fluorescein-conjugated antibody.

Coincubation of the displayed proteins, labeled by fluorescein, and H1 HA, labeled by phycoerythrin, enabled detection of the binding ability of the displayed protein to HA by measuring dual fluorescence by flow cytometry in a high throughput manner (Figure 9).

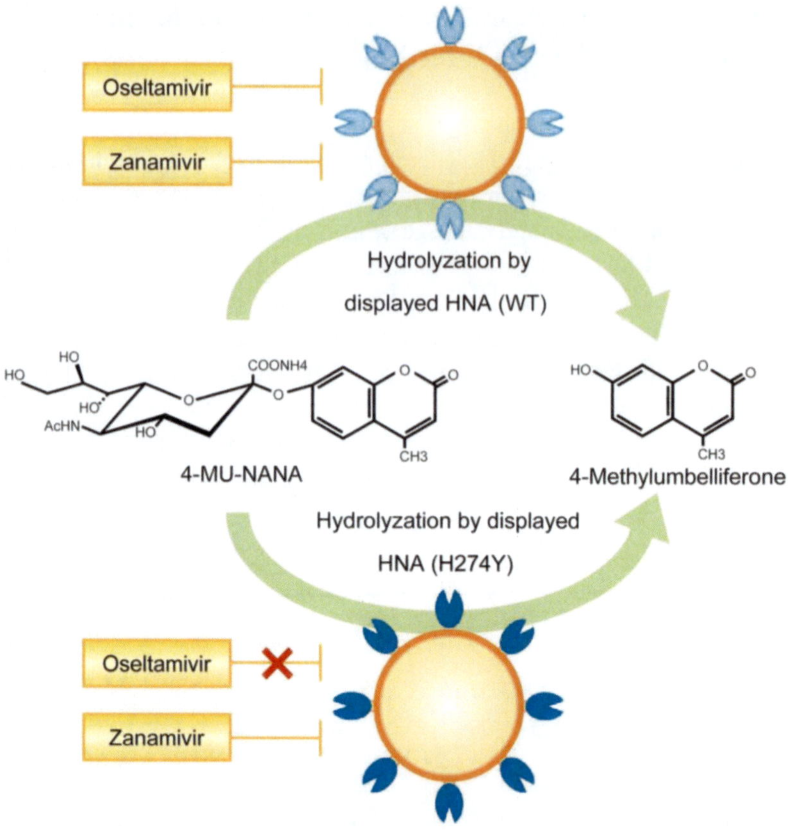

Figure 8. Inhibition assays with displayed WT and mutant (H274Y) HNA [40].

Of the 73 designs displayed on the yeast surface, two proteins, named HB36 and HB80 [42], showed binding activity toward the conserved HA stem region. Because computational design is not perfect due to the numerous approximations involved, affinity maturation of the proteins was performed using a variant library of HB36 and HB80 generated by single site mutation or error-prone polymerase chain reaction (epPCR).

Using yeast displaying the library, the important residues that were needed to improve the affinity were detected, and higher-affinity proteins, named HB36.3 and HB80.3, were obtained. The co-crystal structure of the HB36.3-H1 complex showed the precision of the computer-based design [42]. It was confirmed that HB80.3 had cross-reactivity against several HA subtypes. A complete set of amino acid variants at each position was generated by DNA sequence substitution, and the individual position libraries were then pooled. The displayed proteins that

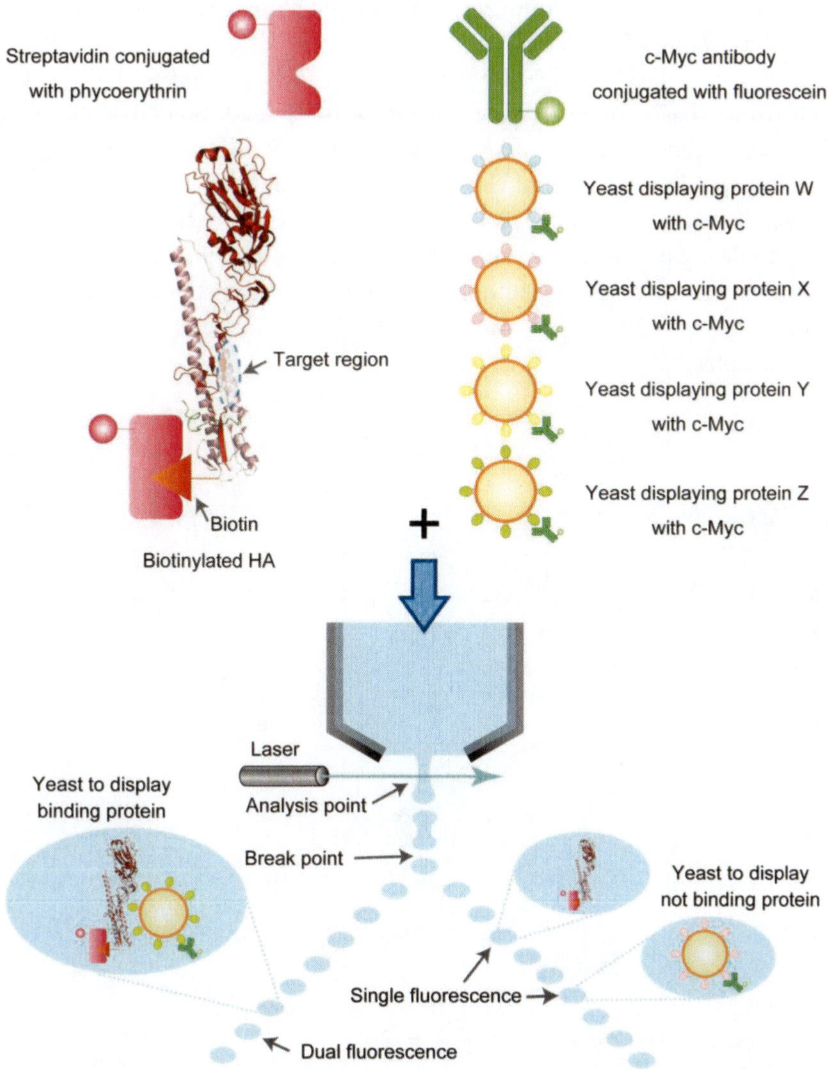

Figure 9. The scheme for screening the designed proteins that bind to HA [42].

bound to either H1 or H5 HA were collected by fluorescence-activated cell sorting (FACS).

Analysis of the enrichment value showed that, the obtained protein, named F-HB80.4, has influenza neutralization activity that is nearly equivalent to that of neutralizing antibodies [43]. These results show that yeast cell surface engineering could be used, in combination with a computational approach, for high-throughput screening of inhibitors.

Detection of the binding site of virus-specific antibodies helps us to understand the basis of their neutralizing activity and potential means of neutralization escape. Analyzing the epitope of HA-specific antibodies, it should be possible to produce a universal vaccine for all HA subtypes.

Although various epitope mapping methods have been reported, it is necessary to develop an easier and more accurate method to quickly determine the epitope of newly discovered neutralizing antibodies against influenza viruses. Yeast cell surface engineering can be applied for fine epitope mapping of antibodies against HA [44].

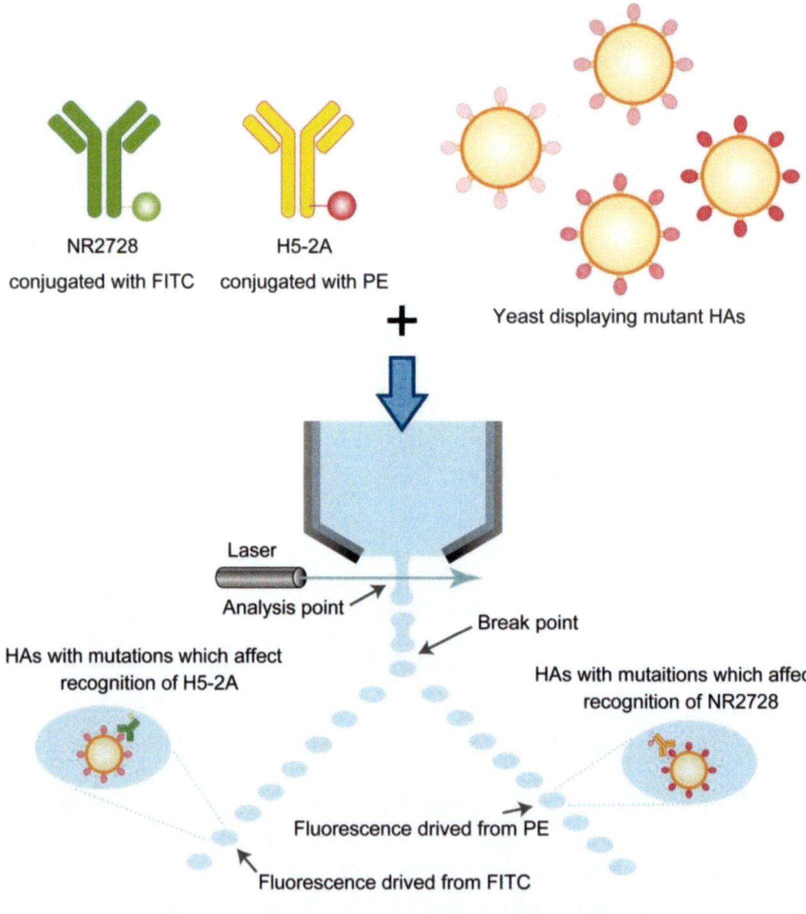

Figure 10. The scheme for fine epitope mapping of antibodies recognizing HA [44].

A yeast displaying library of H5 HA derived from epPCR was used to define the critical residues for recognition of anti-HA monoclonal antibodies (mAbs), such as the H5-2A and NR2728 mAbs. The yeast clones were screened for their lack of binding to H5-2A or NR2728 but retention of binding to other H5-specific antibodies. Then, the binding specificity of the isolated individuals was confirmed by FACS analysis (Figure 10).

It revealed that the H5-2A mAb epitope was located on a single loop buried in the HA1 trimer interface, which is away from the receptor binding site, and that the NR2728 epitope is surface-accessible and contiguous to the receptor binding site.

The fine epitope mapping of anti-HA antibodies using cell surface engineering could further our understanding of the antibody epitopes of highly pathogenic influenza viruses and other emerging influenza strains that may cause the next influenza pandemics.

Traditional vaccination methods against highly pathogenic avian viruses require costly injections to protect poultry. In addition, using current methodology, it takes a long time to produce vaccines. Such time-consuming methods are not sufficient for mounting a rapid response to frequently mutating influenza viruses. Yeast is a promising host for producing antigenic proteins because it glycosylates proteins, which may be important for the generation of neutralizing antibodies.

In addition, the yeast cell wall contains β-glucan, which likely functions an adjuvant. Based on these advantages, yeast cell surface engineering has been used to develop oral vaccines [45-47]. As a test of influenza virus vaccine, HA-displaying yeasts were preliminarily administrated as an oral vaccine [48]. Virus-neutralizing antibodies were detected in the serum of chickens that were orally vaccinated with the H1 HA-displaying yeast. Although the detected antibodies showed a low level of neutralizing activity against influenza virus, optimization of the yeast dosage and the timing of vaccination could improve the production of neutralizing antibodies. This result demonstrated the potential use of HA-displaying yeast as an oral vaccine for the treatment of influenza virus infection.

Conclusion

Various methods have been used to treat influenza virus infections. However, the existing approaches are inadequate to deal with the frequently mutated influenza viruses. In this chapter, we showed that yeast cell surface engineering could be used as a platform for inhibitor screening, antibodies analysis, and vaccines development.

In future studies, cell surface engineering will be a valuable tool for the treatment of frequently mutated viruses, including the influenza virus.

References

[1] Palese, P., Young, J. F. (1982). Variation of influenza A, B, and C viruses. *Science*, 215, 1468-1474.

[2] Fouchier, R. A., Munster, V., Wallensten, A., Bestebroer, T. M., Herfst, S., Smith, D., et al. (2005). Characterization of a novel influenza A virus hemagglutinin subtype (H16) obtained from black-headed gulls. *Journal of Virology,* 79, 2814-2822.

[3] Baker, A. T., Varghese, J. N., Laver, W. G., Air, G. M., Colman, P. M. (1987). Three-dimensional structure of neuraminidase of subtype N9 from an avian influenza virus. *Proteins*, 2, 111-117.

[4] Shinde, V., Bridges, C. B., Uyeki, T. M., Shu, B., Balish, A., Xu, X., et al. (2009). Triple-reassortant swine influenza A (H1) in humans in the United States, 2005–2009. *The New England Journal of Medicine*, 360, 2616-2625.

[5] Nayak, D. P., Balogun, R. A., Yamada, H., Zhou, Z. H., Barman, S. (2009). Influenza virus morphogenesis and budding. *Virus Research*, 143, 147.

[6] Both, G. W., Sleigh, M. J., Cox, N. J., Kendal, A. P. (1983). Antigenic drift in influenza virus H3 hemagglutinin from 1968 to 1980: multiple evolutionary pathways and sequential amino acid changes at key antigenic sites. *Journal of Virology*, 48, 52-60.

[7] Carrat, F., Flahault, A. (2007). Influenza vaccine: the challenge of antigenic drift. *Vaccine*, 25, 6852-6862.

[8] Cox, N. J., Subbarao, K. (2000). Global epidemiology of influenza: past and present. *Annual Review of Medicine*, 51, 407-421.

[9] Holmes, E. C., Ghedin, E., Miller, N., Taylor, J., Bao, Y., St George, K., et al. (2005). Whole-genome analysis of human influenza A virus reveals multiple persistent lineages and reassortment among recent H3N2 viruses. *PLoS Biology*, 3, e300.

[10] Neumann, G., Noda, T., Kawaoka, Y. (2009). Emergence and pandemic potential of swine-origin H1N1 influenza virus. *Nature*, 459, 931-939.

[11] Claas, E. C., Osterhaus, A. D., van Beek, R., De Jong, J. C., Rimmelzwaan, G. F., Senne, D. A., et al. (1998). Human influenza A H5N1 virus related to a highly pathogenic avian influenza virus. *The Lancet,* 351, 472-477.

[12] Wilson, I., Skehel, J., Wiley, D. (1981). Structure of the haemagglutinin membrane glycoprotein of influenza virus at 3 andangst; resolution. *Nature*, 289, 366-373.

[13] Steel, J., Lowen, A. C., Wang, T. T., Yondola, M., Gao, Q., Haye, K., et al. (2010). Influenza virus vaccine based on the conserved hemagglutinin stalk domain. *mBio*, 1, e00018.

[14] Gething, M. J., Doms, R. W., York, D., White, J. (1986). Studies on the mechanism of membrane fusion: site-specific mutagenesis of the hemagglutinin of influenza virus. *The Journal of Cell Biology*, 102, 11-23.

[15] Wiley, D. C., Skehel, J. J. (1987). The structure and function of the hemagglutinin membrane glycoprotein of influenza virus. *Annual Review of Biochemistry,* 56, 365-394.

[16] Sauter, N. K., Bednarski, M. D., Wurzburg, B. A., Hanson, J. E., Whitesides, G. M., Skehel, J. J., et al. (1989). Hemagglutinins from two influenza virus variants bind to sialic acid derivatives with millimolar dissociation constants: a 500-MHz proton nuclear magnetic resonance study. *Biochemistry*, 28, 8388-8396.

[17] Durrer, P., Galli, C., Hoenke, S., Corti, C., Glück, R., Vorherr, T., et al. (1996). H^+-induced membrane insertion of influenza virus hemagglutinin involves the HA2 amino-terminal fusion peptide but not the coiled coil region. *Journal of Biological Chemistry*, 271, 13417-13421.

[18] Cross, K. J., Langley, W. A., Russell, R. J., Skehel, J. J., Steinhauer, D. A. (2009). Composition and functions of the influenza fusion peptide. *Protein and Peptide Letters*, 16, 766-778.

[19] Skehel, J. J., Wiley, D. C. (2000). Receptor binding and membrane fusion in virus entry: the influenza hemagglutinin. *Annual Review of Biochemistry*, 69, 531-569.

[20] Moscona, A. (2005). Neuraminidase inhibitors for influenza. *The New England Journal of Medicine,* 353, 1363-1373.

[21] Xu, R., Zhu, X., McBride, R., Nycholat, C. M., Yu, W., Paulson, J. C., et al. (2012). Functional balance of the hemagglutinin and neuraminidase activities accompanies the emergence of the 2009 H1N1 influenza pandemic. *Journal of Virology*, 86, 9221-9232.

[22] Hay, A. J., Wolstenholme, A. J., Skehel, J. J., Smith, M. H. (1985). The molecular basis of the specific anti-influenza action of amantadine. *The EMBO Journal*, 4, 3021-3024.

[23] Pinto, L. H., Holsinger, L. J., Lamb, R. A. (1992). Influenza virus M2 protein has ion channel activity. *Cell*, 69, 517-528.

[24] Stoof, J. C., Booij, J., Drukarch, B., Wolters, E. C. (1992). The anti-

parkinsonian drug amantadine inhibits the N-methyl-D-aspartic acid-evoked release of acetylcholine from rat neostriatum in a non-competitive way. *European Journal of Pharmacology*, 213, 439-443.

[25] Hayden, F. G., Belshe, R. B., Clover, R. D., Hay, A. J., Oakes, M. G., Soo, W. (1989). Emergence and apparent transmission of rimantadine-resistant influenza A virus in families. *The New England Journal of Medicine,* 321, 1696-1702.

[26] Russell, R. J., Kerry, P. S., Stevens, D. J., Steinhauer, D. A., Martin, S. R., Gamblin, S. J., et al. (2008). Structure of influenza hemagglutinin in complex with an inhibitor of membrane fusion. *Proceedings of the National Academy of Sciences US*, 105, 17736-17741.

[27] Garten, W., Stieneke, A., Shaw, E., Wikstrom, P., Klenk, H. D. (1989). Inhibition of proteolytic activation of influenza virus hemagglutinin by specific peptidyl chloroalkyl ketones. *Virology*, 172, 25-31.

[28] Matsubara, T., Onishi, A., Saito, T., Shimada, A., Inoue, H., Taki, T., et al. (2010). Sialic acid-mimic peptides as hemagglutinin inhibitors for anti-influenza therapy. *Journal of Medicinal Chemistry*, 53, 4441-4449.

[29] Ekiert, D. C., Bhabha, G., Elsliger, M. A., Friesen, R. H., Jongeneelen, M., Throsby, M., et al. (2009). Antibody recognition of a highly conserved influenza virus epitope. *Science*, 324, 246-251.

[30] Von Itzstein, M., Wu, W. Y., Kok, G. B., Pegg, M. S., Dyason, J. C., Jin, B., et al. (1993). Rational design of potent sialidase-based inhibitors of influenza virus replication. *Nature*, 363, 418-423.

[31] Kim, C. U., Lew, W., Williams, M. A., Liu, H., Zhang, L., Swaminathan, S., et al. (1997). Influenza neuraminidase inhibitors possessing a novel hydrophobic interaction in the enzyme active site: design, synthesis, and structural analysis of carbocyclic sialic acid analogues with potent anti-influenza activity. *Journal of the American Chemical Society,* 119, 681-690.

[32] Ives, J. A., Carr, J. A., Mendel, D. B., Tai, C. Y., Lambkin, R., Kelly, L., et al. (2002). The H274Y mutation in the influenza A/H1N1 neuraminidase active site following oseltamivir phosphate treatment leave virus severely compromised both *in vitro* and *in vivo*. *Antiviral Research*, 55, 307-317.

[33] Staschke, K. A., Colacino, J. M., Baxter, A. J., Air, G. M., Bansal, A., Hornback, W. J., et al. (1995). Molecular basis for the resistance of influenza viruses to 4-guanidino-Neu5Ac2en. *Virology*, 214, 642-646.

[34] Babu, Y. S., Chand, P., Bantia, S., Kotian, P., Dehghani, A., El-Kattan, Y., et al. (2000). BCX-1812 (RWJ-270201): discovery of a novel, highly potent, orally active, and selective influenza neuraminidase inhibitor through structure-based drug design. *Journal of Medicinal Chemistry*, 43, 3482-

3486.

[35] Yamamoto, T., Kumazawa, H., Inami, K., Teshima, T., Shiba, T. (1992). Syntheses of sialic-acid isomers with inhibitory activity against neuraminidase. *Tetrahedron Letters*, 33, 5791-5794.

[36] Gubareva, L. V., Kaiser, L., Hayden, F. G. (2000). Influenza virus neuraminidase inhibitors. *The Lancet*, 355, 827-835.

[37] Bantia, S., Arnold, C. S., Parker, C. D., Upshaw, R., Chand, P. (2006). Anti-influenza virus activity of peramivir in mice with single intramuscular injection. *Antiviral Research*, 69, 39-45.

[38] Ueda, M. (2011). Revolutionary protein engineering using molecular display. *Protein Engineering: Design, Selection and Applications* (Nova Science Publisher), 73-80.

[39] Fushimi, T., Miura, N., Shintani, H., Tsunoda, H., Kuroda, K., Ueda, M. (2013). Mutant firefly luciferases with improved specific activity and dATP discrimination constructed by yeast cell surface engineering. *Applied Microbiology and Biotechnology*, 97, 4003-4011.

[40] Shigemori, T., Nagayama, M., Yamada, J., Miura, N., Yongkiettrakul, S., Kuroda, K., et al. (2013). Construction of a convenient system for easily screening inhibitors of mutated influenza virus neuraminidases. *FEBS Open Bio*, 3, 484-489.

[41] Kortemme, T., Joachimiak, L. A., Bullock, A. N., Schuler, A. D., Stoddard, B. L., Baker, D. (2004). Computational redesign of protein-protein interaction specificity. *Nature Structural and Molecular Biology*, 11, 371-379.

[42] Fleishman, S. J., Whitehead, T. A., Ekiert, D. C., Dreyfus, C., Corn, J. E., Strauch, E. M., et al. (2011). Computational design of proteins targeting the conserved stem region of influenza hemagglutinin. *Science*, 332, 816-821.

[43] Whitehead, T. A., Chevalier, A., Song, Y., Dreyfus, C., Fleishman, S. J., De Mattos, C., et al. (2012). Optimization of affinity, specificity and function of designed influenza inhibitors using deep sequencing. *Nature Biotechnology*, 30, 543-548.

[44] Han, T., Sui, J., Bennett, A. S., Liddington, R. C., Donis, R. O., Zhu, Q., et al. (2011). Fine epitope mapping of monoclonal antibodies against hemagglutinin of a highly pathogenic H5N1 influenza virus using yeast surface display. *Biochemical and Biophysical Research Communications,* 409, 253-259.

[45] Tamaru, Y., Ohtsuka, M., Kato, K., Manabe, S., Kuroda, K., Sanada, M., et al. (2006). Application of the arming system for the expression of the 380R antigen from red sea bream iridovirus (RSIV) on the surface of yeast cells: a

first step for the development of an oral vaccine. *Biotechnology Progress*, 22, 949-953.

[46] Shibasaki, S., Ueda, M. (2010). Development of yeast molecular display systems focused on therapeutic proteins, enzymes, and foods: functional analysis of proteins and its application to bioconversion. *Recent Patent Biotechnology,* 4, 198-213.

[47] Shibasaki, S., Aoki, W., Nomura, T., Miyoshi, A., Tafuku, S., Sewaki, T., et al. (2013). An oral vaccine against candidiasis generated by a yeast molecular display system. *Pathogens and Disease*, 69, 262-268.

[48] Wasilenko, J. L., Sarmento, L., Spatz, S., Pantin-Jackwood, M. (2010). Cell surface display of highly pathogenic avian influenza virus hemagglutinin on the surface of *Pichia pastoris* cells using alpha-agglutinin for production of oral vaccines. *Biotechnology Progress*, 26, 542-547.

In: Influenza and RNA Viruses
Editor: R. H. Bishop, pp. 111-122
ISBN: 978-1-63321-799-7

Chapter 6

SALIVIRUS/KLASSEVIRUS: AN EMERGING VIRUS ASSOCIATED WITH PAEDIATRIC DIARRHEA/ACUTE FLACCID PARALYSIS AND ENVIRONMENTAL CONTAMINATION

Masaaki Kitajima[1,*], Eiji Haramoto[2] and Charles P. Gerba[3]
[1]Center for Environmental Sensing and Modeling,
Singapore-MIT Alliance for Research and Technology, Singapore
[2]International Research Center for River Basin Environment,
University of Yamanashi, Yamanashi, Japan
[3]Department of Soil, Water and Environmental Science,
The University of Arizona, Tucson, Arizona, US

Abstract

Salivirus and klassevirus, possessing a positive-sense polyadenylated single-stranded RNA genome, are novel members of the family *Picornaviridae* and most closely related to Aichi virus of the genus *Kobuvirus*. Both salivirus and klassevirus were first described in 2009; salivirus was discovered in the feces of children with non-polio acute flaccid paralysis (AFP) in Nigeria (Stool Aichi-LIke virus), whereas klassevirus was found in the feces of children with gastroenteritis in the United States and Australia as well as in a sewage sample collected in Spain (Kobu-Like virus Associated with Stool and SEwage).

* E-mail address: kitajima@smart.mit.edu (Corresponding Author).

Salivirus is genetically indistinguishable from klassevirus, and these viruses are currently classified into the novel genus, *Salivirus*. Salivirus/klassevirus has been identified in the feces of patients in Asian, European, and South American continents as well, suggesting its worldwide distribution. Recent studies also detected salivirus/klassevirus in wastewater, river water, and biosolids, in Asian, European, and American continents. These recent findings have suggested that salivirus and klassevirus are emerging viral pathogens associated with gastroenteritis or non-polio AFP in infants and environmental transmission is likely. Further clinical and environmental studies are needed to better understand their prevalence, distribution, molecular epidemiology, and significance to public health.

1. Introduction

Salivirus and klassevirus, possessing a positive-sense polyadenylated single-stranded RNA genome, are novel members of the family *Picornaviridae* and most closely related to Aichi virus of the genus *Kobuvirus*. Both salivirus and klassevirus were first described in 2009. Salivirus was discovered in the feces of children with non-polio acute flaccid paralysis (AFP) in Nigeria (Stool Aichi-LIke virus) (Li et al., 2009). Two independent research groups reported the discovery of klassevirus at almost the same time. Holtz et al. (2009) reported the identification of klassevirus in the feces of children with gastroenteritis in the United States and Australia as well as in a sewage sample collected in Spain (Kobu-Like virus Associated with Stool and SEwage) (Holtz et al., 2009). Greninger et al. (2009) also reported the discovery of klassevirus in stool from infants from Northern California, United States, and carried out complete genome analysis. Salivirus is genetically indistinguishable from klassevirus, and these viruses are currently classified into the novel genus, *Salivirus* according to the *Picornaviridae* Study Group of the International Committee on Taxonomy of Viruses (ICTV) (http://www.picornastudygroup.com/).

Salivirus/klassevirus has been identified in the feces of gastroenteritis or non-polio AFP patients in Asian, African, European, and North and South American continents (Greninger et al., 2009, 2010; Han et al., 2010; Holtz et al., 2009; Li et al., 2009; Nielsen et al., 2013; Nix et al., 2013; Shan et al., 2010), suggesting its worldwide distribution. Recent environmental studies also revealed the occurrence of salivirus/klassevirus in the environments, such as wastewater, river water, and biosolids, in Asian, European, and North and South American continents (Bibby & Peccia, 2013; Calgua et al., 2013; Han et al., 2014; Haramoto et al., 2013; Haramoto & Otagiri, 2013; Holtz et al., 2009; Kitajima et al., in press; Ng et al., 2012), which indicates that these viruses are disseminated in the environment worldwide. This chapter focuses on salivirus/klassevirus as an emerging RNA virus associated with paediatric diarrhea/non-polio AFP and environmental occurrence.

2. Salivirus/Klassevirus from Diarrhea/Non-polio AFP Patients

Detection of salivirus/klassevirus in clinical samples from diarrhea/non-polio AFP patients is summarized in Table 1. The virus has been detected in up to 8.8% in patients with gastroenteritis and a seroprevalence of 6.8%.

Holtz et al. (2009) first reported the detection and genomic characterization of a novel picornavirus, klassevirus, in a stool specimen collected in Australia in 1984 from a child with acute diarrhea, by combination of mass sequencing with 454 pyrosequencing technology, reverse transcription-polymerase chain reaction (RT-PCR), 5' random amplification of cDNA ends (RACE), and 3' RACE. Phylogenetic analysis of the genome demonstrated that this virus was highly divergent from all previously described picornaviruses and its closest relatives appeared to be the members of the genus *Kobuvirus*, which includes Aichi virus, bovine kobuvirus, and porcine kobuvirus (Holtz et al., 2009). The prevalence of klassevirus among paediatric patients with acute diarrhea was subsequently investigated by RT-PCR, and one (0.3%) out of 340 stool specimens from St. Louis, US was tested positive for klassevirus (Holtz et al., 2009). In parallel, another study also identified klassevirus by performing 454 pyrosequencing on a pool of 141 paediatric gastroenteritis stool samples from Northern California, US, that were previously found to be negative for known diarrheal viruses (Greninger et al., 2009). Independent screening of each of the pooled stool specimens was subsequently performed, and the virus was identified in two children who were asymptomatic at the time of sample collection with viral RNA level of 1-5 × 10^7 copies/1mL-stool as determined by SYBR Green-based quantitative PCR (qPCR) (Greninger et al., 2009).

Li et al. (2009) reported the discovery and genomic characterization of a similar picornavirus, salivirus, in stool specimens from two of 95 Nigerian children suffering from non-polio AFP. Divergent strains of salivirus were identified in 18 stool samples from Nigeria, Tunisia, Nepal, and US via RT-nested PCR. All stool samples tested positive were from diseased (non-polio AFP or gastroenteritis) individuals (N = 377), whereas none of the samples from healthy control (N = 288) were positive for salivirus. Shan et al. (2010) also reported that salivirus was found in a higher proportion of cases in Chinese children with

Table 1. Detection of salivirus/klassevirus genomes or antibodies in clinical samples from diarrheal/AFP patients

Symptom	Sample	Patient age[1]	Country	Method	Detection ratio	Reference
Diarrhea/ Gastroenteritis	Stool	<5 yrs	Australia	NGS[2] mass sequencing, RT-PCR	NGS: 1/1 (100%), PCR: 0/143 (0%)	(Holtz et al., 2009)
	Stool	Paediatric	US (Missouri)	RT-PCR	1/340 (0.3%)	(Holtz et al., 2009)
	Stool	Paediatric	US (California)	NGS mass sequencing, RT-PCR	NGS: 1/141 (0.7%), PCR: 2/751 (0.2%)	(Greninger et al., 2009)
	Stool	Adult travellers	Nepal	RT-nested PCR	8/92 (8.7%)	(Li et al., 2009)
	Stool	N.A.	US (Minnesota)	RT-nested PCR	2/96 (2.1%)	(Li et al., 2009)
	Stool	2~6 years	China	RT-nested PCR-cloning-sequencing	9/216 (4.2%)	(Shan et al., 2010)
	Stool	<5 yrs	India	RT-PCR	25/416 (6.0%)	(Greninger et al., 2010)
	Serum	1 day ~ 79 yrs	US (Missouri)	ELISA	24/353 (6.8%)	(Greninger et al., 2010)
	Stool	<17 years	South Korea	RT-nested PCR-sequencing	26/294 (8.8%)	(Han et al., 2010)
	Stool[2]	<15 mo	Denmark	RT-qPCR	Patients: 8/386 (2.1%), Control: 1/1,007 (0.1%)	(Nielsen et al., 2013)
Non-polio AFP	Stool	0.5 mo ~ 15 yrs	Nigeria	NGS mass sequencing, RT-nested PCR	NGS: 2/95 (2.1%), PCR: 5/93(5.4%)	(Li et al., 2009)
	Stool	0.5 mo ~ 15 yrs	Tunisia	RT-nested PCR	3/96 (3.1%)	(Li et al., 2009)
	Stool[3]	1~21 yrs	Bolivia	RT-qPCR	Patients: 1/49 (2.0%), Control: 0/32 (0%)	(Nix et al., 2013)

[1]N.A., not available. [2]NGS, next-generation sequencing, [3]Control samples (i.e., stool specimens from healthy individuals) were also included in the study.

Table 2. Detection of salivirus/klassevirus in environmental samples

Sample	Country	Method	Detection ratio	Concentration (copies/L)[1]	Reference
Raw sewage	Spain	RT-PCR	1/1 (100%)	N.A.	(Holtz et al., 2009)
	Nepal, Thailand, Nigeria, US (California)	Metagenomics, RT-PCR	2/4 (50%)	N.A.	(Ng et al., 2012)
	Japan	RT-nested PCR, RT-qPCR	2C-nested: 5/14 (36%); 3D-nested: 4/14 (29%); VP0/VP1-nested: 0/14 (0%); 5’ UTR-nested: 2/14 (14%); qPCR: 13/14 (93%)	3.7×10^5–9.7×10^6	(Haramoto and Otagiri, 2013; Haramoto et al., 2013)
	South Korea	RT-nested PCR	8/14 (57%)	N.A.	(Han et al., 2014)
	US (Arizona)	RT-nested PCR, RT-qPCR	Nested: 5/24 (21%); qPCR: 11/24 (46%)	2.32×10^3–1.80×10^5	(Kitajima et al., in press)
Treated sewage	Japan	RT-nested PCR, RT-qPCR	2C-nested: 1/14 (7%); 3D-nested: 3/14 (21%); VP0/VP1-nested: 0/14 (0%); 5’ UTR-nested: 1/14 (7%); qPCR: 4/14 (29%)	1.6×10^4–7.1×10^4	(Haramoto and Otagiri, 2013; Haramoto et al., 2013)
	US (Arizona)	RT-nested PCR, RT-qPCR	Nested: 2/24 (8%); qPCR: 11/24 (46%)	6.95×10^2–2.46×10^4	(Kitajima et al., in press)
Sewage sludge	US	Metagenomics	11/12 (92%)	N.A.	(Bibby and Peccia, 2013)
River water	Japan	RT-qPCR	9/56 (16%)	1.7×10^4–2.7×10^5	(Haramoto et al., 2013)
	Spain, Brazil	RT-nested PCR	Spain: 0/6 (0%); Brazil: 2/6 (33%)	N.A.	(Calgua et al., 2013)

[1]Range of salivirus/klassevirus-RNA concentration in positive samples; N.A., not available.

diarrhea (9/216, 4.2%) compared to asymptomatic children (0/96, 0%). Klassevirus was further identified in children with gastroenteritis in South Korea (26/294, 8.8%), suggesting possible association between this virus and gastroenteritis (Han et al., 2010). A search for antibodies against klassevirus protease 3C in a cohort of 353 patients in St. Louis, US, revealed a seroprevalence of 6.8% (24/353), suggesting that klassevirus infection and replication occur in humans (Greninger et al., 2010).

Nielsen et al. (2013) reported that salivirus was detected in one (0.1%) out of 1,007 samples from healthy individuals and 8 (2.1%) out of 386 samples from gastroenteritis patients in Denmark, suggesting that salivirus may be associated with and a possible cause of paediatric gastroenteritis. In addition, Nix et al. (2013) reported the detection of salivirus from one (2.0%) out of 51 stool samples from AFP patients in Bolivia.

3. Salivirus/Klassevirus in the Environment

Since sewage or sewage-contaminated waters may contain viruses shed from all individuals within a catchment/service area regardless of their symptoms, testing of these waters could be an effective approach to determine the circulation of viruses within a population and in addition to obtaining sequence information of the circulating strains; especially for emerging viruses or viruses rarely identified in clinical cases, including salivirus/klassevirus. Several studies have reported the detection of salivirus/klassevirus in environmental samples, as summarized in Table 2.

Detection of salivirus/klassevirus in an environmental sample was first reported by Holtz et al. (2009). In this study, the virus was detected by RT-PCR assays targeting 2C, 3D, and VP0/VP1 regions in a raw sewage sample in Spain. Subsequently, salivirus genomes were identified in raw sewage samples collected from Nepal and Thailand by viral metagenomics (Ng et al., 2012). Haramoto and Otagiri (2013) investigated the seasonal occurrence and genetic diversity of salivirus/klassevirus in Japanese wastewater collected over a 14-month period. This study utilized three RT-nested PCR assays targeting different genomic regions, namely, 2C, 3D, and VP0/VP1, and found salivirus/klassevirus in seven (50%) raw sewage and four (29%) secondary-treated sewage samples. Haramoto et al. (2013) subsequently examined the prevalence of salivirus/klassevirus in wastewater and river water in Japan using a newly developed RT-qPCR assay targeting 5’ untranslated region (UTR) and reported that this virus was frequently detected in wastewater and river water samples with a concentration of 1.6×10^4

to 9.7 × 10^6 copies/L, providing the first quantitative data on the occurrence of this virus in environmental water. Although there have been no reports of salivirus/klassevirus detection in clinical samples in Japan, these findings suggest that salivirus/klassevirus infection occurs in Japan, probably throughout the year. Haramoto et al. (2013) also demonstrated that wastewater treatment was capable of reducing the virus by >3 $\log_{10}$, which is usually greater than that of other human enteric viruses, such as adenoviruses and noroviruses - this may explain the lower detection frequency in river water samples observed in this study. The presence of klassevirus in raw sewage in South Korea has been also in 8/14 (57%) using RT-nested PCR (Han et al., 2014).

More recently, we reported the detection and genetic analysis of salivirus/klassevirus in wastewater at two treatment plants in Arizona, US, using RT-qPCR and RT-nested PCR-cloning-sequencing (Kitajima et al., in press). Salivirus/klassevirus was detected in 11 (46%) out of 24 samples in both influent and effluent wastewater, with a maximum concentration of 2.28 × 10^5 and 2.46 × 10^4 copies/L, respectively. Based on the sequencing analysis, a total of 49 salivirus/klassevirus sequences were identified, which demonstrates the diversity of virus strains infecting humans. These findings on the occurrence of salivirus/klassevirus suggest that this virus occurs in sewage-contaminated waters and is capable of waterborne transmission and waterborne viral infection/diseases.

4. Ongoing Progress and Future Study Directions

Recent advancements in next-generation sequencing technology and metagenomics have opened the door to discovery of new human viruses, particularly in stool specimens, such as the recently characterized new picornaviruses, including salivirus/klassevirus. The genome of salivirus/klassevirus is approximately 8.0 kbp in length, which is comprised of a 5' UTR

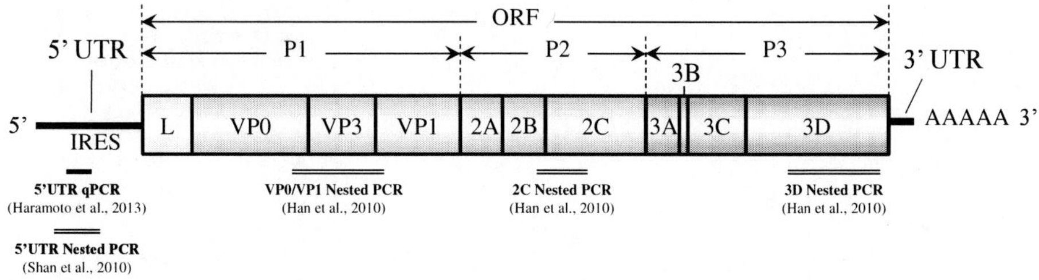

Figure 1. Genome organization of salivirus/klassevirus and target locations of diagnostic PCR assays.

region with an internal ribosomal entry site (IRES), a large open reading frame (ORF) of approximately 7.1 kbp encoding a putative protein precursor, and a 3' UTR region (Greninger et al., 2009; Li et al., 2009), as shown in Figure 1. The polyprotein starts with a leader (L) peptide, followed by structural proteins (VP0, VP3, and VP1) and non-structural proteins P2 (2A, 2B, and 2C) and P3 (3A, 3B, 3C, and 3D).

Based on the sequencing data, several RT-PCR and RT-nested PCR assays targeting the conserved nucleotide sequences in the 5' UTR, 2C, 3D, and VP0/VP3/VP1 regions of salivirus/klassevirus have been developed (Greninger et al., 2009; Han et al., 2010; Holtz et al., 2009; Li et al., 2009; Shan et al., 2010); in addition, a salivirus/klassevirus-specific RT-qPCR assay targeting the 5' UTR was recently developed based on alignment of 16 salivirus/klassevirus sequences obtained from clinical and environmental (wastewater) samples (Haramoto et al., 2013) (See Figure 1).

The developed qPCR assay allowed for the detection of as little as one copy of plasmid DNA, demonstrating a comparable sensitivity to conventional nested PCR for plasmid DNA amplification (Haramoto et al., 2013). The development of salivirus/klassevirus-specific RT-nested PCR and RT-qPCR will facilitate further

(A)

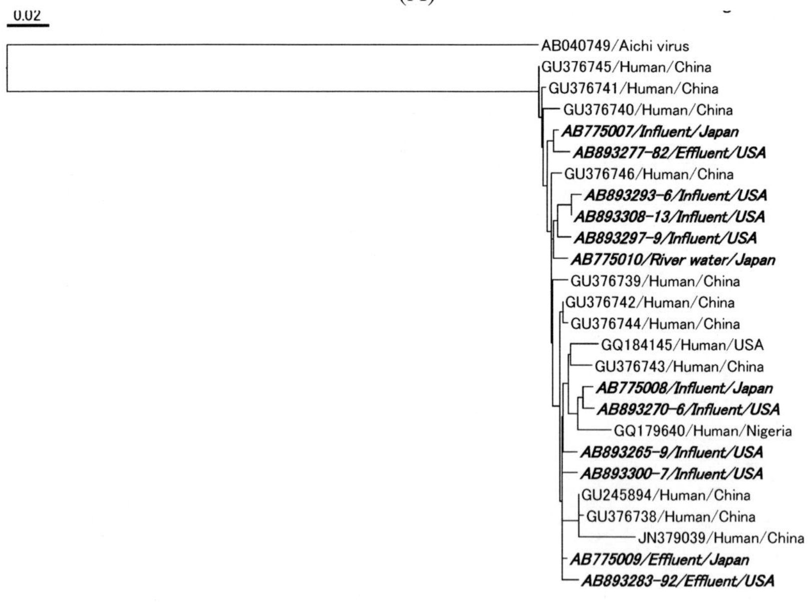

Figure 2. Continued on next page.

(B)

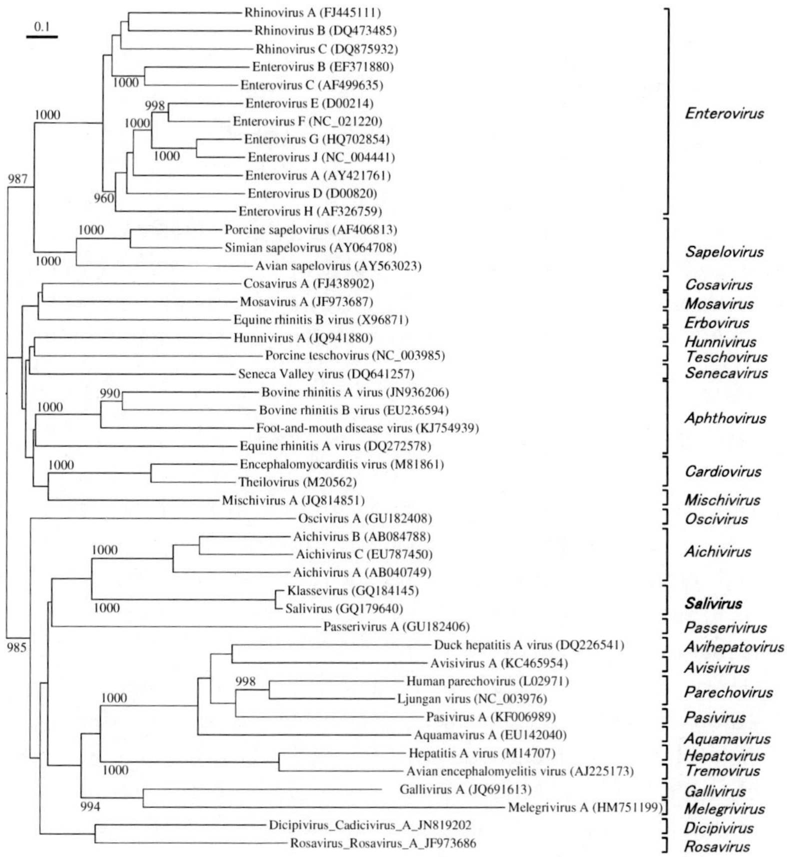

Figure 2. (A) Phylogenetic relationship of salivirus/klassevirus with representative species from each picornavirus genus, based on amino acid similarity of P1 region using neighbour-joining method. (B) Phylogenetic tree for salivirus/klassevirus strains based on the 5' UTR gene sequences. Strains shown in *italic* are salivirus/klassevirus strains identified in environmental samples. The scale represents amino acid (A) or nucleotide (B) substitutions per site.

investigation on the prevalence of this virus in clinical stool specimens and environmental samples. Although the previous studies have suggested that salivirus/klassevirus is associated with gastroenteritis or non-polio AFP, some studies reported the detection of this virus from healthy individuals, indicating that not all salivirus/klassevirus infections are associated with human diseases.

More epidemiological studies with sufficient number of healthy/asymptomatic specimens are needed to reach a definitive conclusion on the association of this virus with gastroenteritis or non-polio AFP.

Further environmental studies are required to better understand the prevalence and behavior of this emerging virus in various types of water worldwide. It is also essential to establish a cell culture infectivity assay for this virus to assess its persistence in the environments and susceptibility to disinfectants. In epidemiological and environmental studies, it is recommended to target other recently characterized picornaviruses as well (e.g., Saffold virus, cosavirus, and Aichi virus), considering their potential to cause human diseases (Nielsen et al., 2013; Nix et al., 2013; Tapparel et al., 2013) and previous findings on their prevalence in the environment (Haramoto & Otagiri, 2014; Kitajima et al., 2011).

Conclusion

Salivirus/klassevirus was recently discovered from feces of paediatric gastroenteritis and non-polio AFP patients through a next-generation mass sequencing strategy. Subsequently, this virus was also identified in the environment, such as wastewater, river water, and biosolids. These findings have suggested that salivirus/klassevirus is an emerging viral pathogen associated with gastroenteritis or non-polio AFP in infants and environmental contamination. Accumulation of nucleotide sequence data enabled design and development of several molecular diagnostic assays, including RT-nested PCR and RT-qPCR, for specific detection and quantification of salivirus/klassevirus genomes in various types of samples. Further clinical and environmental studies utilizing these recently developed molecular tools are needed to better understand their prevalence, distribution, molecular epidemiology, and significance in human enteric diseases and public health.

References

Bibby, K., Peccia, J., 2013. Identification of viral pathogen diversity in sewage sludge by metagenome analysis. *Environ. Sci. Technol.* 47, 1945–1951.

Calgua, B., Fumian, T., Rusiñol, M., Rodriguez-Manzano, J., Mbayed, V.A., Bofill-Mas, S., Miagostovich, M., Girones, R., 2013. Detection and quantification of classic and emerging viruses by skimmed-milk flocculation and PCR in river water from two geographical areas. *Water Res.* 47, 2797–810.

Greninger, A.L., Holtz, L., Kang, G., Ganem, D., Wang, D., DeRisi, J.L., 2010. Serological evidence of human klassevirus infection. *Clin. Vaccine Immunol.* 17, 1584–8.

Greninger, A.L., Runckel, C., Chiu, C.Y., Haggerty, T., Parsonnet, J., Ganem, D., Derisi, J.L., 2009. The complete genome of klassevirus – a novel picornavirus in pediatric stool. *Virol. J.* 9, 1–9.

Han, T.-H., Kim, C.H., Chung, J.Y., Park, S.H., Hwang, E.S., 2010. Klassevirus infection in children, South Korea. *Emerg. Infect. Dis.* 16, 1623–5.

Han, T.-H., Kim, S.-C., Kim, S.-T., Chung, C.-H., Chung, J.-Y., 2014. Detection of norovirus genogroup IV, klassevirus, and pepper mild mottle virus in sewage samples in South Korea. *Arch. Virol.* 159, 457–63.

Haramoto, E., Kitajima, M., Otagiri, M., 2013. Development of a reverse transcription-quantitative polymerase chain reaction assay for detection of salivirus/klassevirus. *Appl. Environ. Microbiol.* 79, 3529–3532.

Haramoto, E., Otagiri, M., 2013. Prevalence and genetic diversity of klassevirus in wastewater in Japan. *Food Environ. Virol.* 5, 46–51.

Haramoto, E., Otagiri, M., 2014. Occurrence of human cosavirus in wastewater and river water in Japan. *Food Environ. Virol.* 6, 62–66.

Holtz, L.R., Finkbeiner, S.R., Zhao, G., Kirkwood, C.D., Girones, R., Pipas, J.M., Wang, D., 2009. Klassevirus 1, a previously undescribed member of the family Picornaviridae, is globally widespread. *Virol. J.* 6, 86.

Kitajima, M., Haramoto, E., Phanuwan, C., Katayama, H., 2011. Prevalence and genetic diversity of Aichi viruses in wastewater and river water in Japan. *Appl. Environ. Microbiol.* 77, 2184–2187.

Kitajima, M., Haramoto, E., Rachmadi, A.T., Iker, B.C., Gerba, C.P., in press. Quantification and genetic analysis of salivirus/klassevirus in wastewater in Arizona, USA. *Food Environ. Virol.*

Li, L., Victoria, J., Kapoor, A., Blinkova, O., Wang, C., Babrzadeh, F., Mason, C.J., Pandey, P., Triki, H., Bahri, O., Oderinde, B.S., Baba, M.M., Bukbuk, D.N., Besser, J.M., Bartkus, J.M., Delwart, E.L., 2009. A novel picornavirus associated with gastroenteritis. *J. Virol.* 83, 12002–6.

Ng, T.F.F., Marine, R., Wang, C., Simmonds, P., Kapusinszky, B., Bodhidatta, L., Oderinde, B.S., Wommack, K.E., Delwart, E., 2012. High variety of known and new RNA and DNA viruses of diverse origins in untreated sewage. *J. Virol.* 86, 12161–75.

Nielsen, A.C.Y., Gyhrs, M.L., Nielsen, L.P., Pedersen, C., Böttiger, B., 2013. Gastroenteritis and the novel picornaviruses aichi virus, cosavirus, saffold virus, and salivirus in young children. *J. Clin. Virol.* 57, 239–42.

Nix, W.A., Khetsuriani, N., Peñaranda, S., Maher, K., Venczel, L., Cselkó, Z., Freire, M.C., Cisterna, D., Lema, C.L., Rosales, P., Rodriguez, J.R., Rodriguez, W., Halkyer, P., Ronveaux, O., Pallansch, M. a, Oberste, M.S., 2013. Diversity of picornaviruses in rural Bolivia. *J. Gen. Virol.* 94, 2017–28.

Shan, T., Wang, C., Cui, L., Yu, Y., Delwart, E., Zhao, W., Zhu, C., Lan, D., Dai, X., Hua, X., 2010. Picornavirus salivirus/klassevirus in children with diarrhea, China. *Emerg. Infect. Dis.* 16, 1303–1305.

Tapparel, C., Siegrist, F., Petty, T.J., Kaiser, L., 2013. Picornavirus and enterovirus diversity with associated human diseases. Infect. *Genet. Evol.* 14, 282–93.

INDEX

A

B

C

D

E

F

G

L

M

N

O

P

Q

R

S

T

U

V

W

Y